Dysphasia

Professional Guidance for Family and Patient

CHARLES VAN RIPER, editor   *Foundations of Speech Pathology Series*

Prentice-Hall Foundations of Speech Pathology Series

PRENTICE-HALL INTERNATIONAL, INC., *London*
PRENTICE-HALL OF AUSTRALIA, PTY. LTD., *Sydney*
PRENTICE-HALL OF CANADA, LTD., *Toronto*
PRENTICE-HALL OF INDIA PRIVATE LTD., *New Delhi*
PRENTICE-HALL OF JAPAN, INC., *Tokyo*

Dysphasia

Professional Guidance for Family and Patient

WITHDRAWN

McKenzie Buck

Head, Speech Pathology and Research
Portland Center for Hearing and Speech
Department of Otolaryngology
University of Oregon Medical School

(Chapter I by
Richard P. Schmidt
Associate Dean and Chief of Staff
College of Medicine
University of Florida)

Prentice-Hall, Inc., *Englewood Cliffs, N. J.*

To My Family

This book, in itself an almost impossible task for one who himself has known dysphasia, has been made possible primarily through the understanding and patience and loving care of my wife, Bette, the sincere devotion of my son, Bill, and affectionate enthusiasm of my daughter, Judy.

In Appreciation

I wish also to express my great appreciation to Dr. Richard P. Schmidt, one of the best neurologists I know, for the major contribution he has given in writing the first chapter of this book.

editor's note

THE SET OF VOLUMES WHICH CONSTITUTES THE *Foundations of Speech Pathology* is designed to serve as the nucleus of a professional library, both for students of speech pathology and audiology and for the practicing clinician. Each individual text in the series is written by an author whose authority has long been recognized in his field. Each author has done his utmost to provide the basic information concerning the speech or hearing disorders covered in his book. Our new profession needs new tools, good ones, to be used not once but many times. The flood of new information already upon us requires organization if it is to be assimilated and if it is to help us solve the many different professional problems which beset us. This series provides that essential organization.

One of the unifying and outstanding features of all the volumes in this series is the use of search items. In addition to providing the core of information concerning his subject, each author has indicated clearly other sources having significance for the topic being discussed. The reader is urged to explore, to search, and to discover —and the trails are charted. In so rapidly changing a profession as ours, we cannot afford to remain content with what we have been taught. We must learn to continue learning.

Although each individual volume in this series is complete unto itself, the instructor should welcome the opportunity presented by the *Foundations of Speech Pathology* to combine several volumes to form the basic structure of the course he teaches. They may also be used as collateral readings. These short but comprehensive books give the instructor a thoroughly flexible teaching tool. But the primary aim of the authors of these texts has been the creation of a basic library for all of our students and professional workers. In this series we have sought to provide a common fund of knowledge to help unify and serve our new profession.

contents

chapter IV

chapter V

Richard P. Schmidt, M.D.

INTRODUCTION

THIS CHAPTER DEALS WITH THE FUNCTION OF THE CENTRAL NERVOUS system in speech and language. It is principally concerned with the aphasic disturbances caused by disease processes in parts of the brain, particularly the cerebral cortex. The orientation is derived from clinical neurology. Our information about aphasia comes largely from empiric clinical observation, and although we have accumulated a considerable body of knowledge, we are still at the very frontiers of understanding the intricate activities of the nervous system and the way they affect our behavior.

Speech, the most characteristically human form of behavior, is ultimately controlled by the nervous system. Speech makes use of

1 *neurological dysfunctions*

learning, thinking, and emotion, which are easier for us to understand in psychological than in neurological terms. Most of the neurological information about speech and language has come from studying the correlations between the defects observed in aphasic patients and the localization and extent of lesions in the brain. These correlations have significance, but they do not mean that we thoroughly understand the fundamental neural processes that underly them.

Speech and language are considerably complex. They are produced by a series of reflexes, coordinated movements, and sensations, including those of higher and lower orders of nervous integration. No other animal species has developed linguistic symbols as components of their utterance, even though communication does take place in subhuman species. Speech requires smooth interaction among the many muscles that control our breathing, vocal cords, throat, tongue, lips, and jaw. Speaking also requires the check-and-balance systems that receive continuous feedback from our sense organs. Additional meanings are given to speech by gestures, facial expression, and body postures. All these components of speech are ultimately controlled by the brain.

This chapter deals with the highest level of integration, which, when disturbed, gives rise to dysphasia and associated disturbances. This level of integration is primarily a function of the mantle of nerve cells at the surface of the brain, the cerebral cortex. When parts of the cerebral cortex are diseased as for example, from a stroke, the ability to use language symbols may be impaired or lost, thus limiting communication with others and further disturbing the inner use of language symbols in thought or emotional control. The form or manifestation that this limitation takes depends to a great extent on the area of the brain that is damaged, on how much brain tissue is involved, and also on other factors such as age and psychological adaptiveness. In some patients, difficulty in expression may predominate with relative retention of comprehension. On the other hand, the ability to say *words* may not be lost, but comprehension, syntax, and grammar may be so disordered as to render communication ineffective. The person who becomes dysphasic usually has other manifestations of his illness such as weakness of the right side of the body, loss of sensation, or disturbances of vision. He may also lose the ability to relate his body to the environment about him or to relate parts of his body to himself. The body image, the core of self, may be distorted. He may be unable to recognize the significance of sounds. He may lose the ability to correlate the visual impression of an object with its function, or its name. Some patients cannot even recognize their own images in the mirror. Similarly, he may lose the ability to perform certain learned acts such as reading, writing, or playing bridge.

These impairments and deficits are not to be equated with deafness, blindness, or paralysis as such. They represent an inability to make use of the brain for symbolic constructions and correlations. The disturbances of recognition or appreciation of symbols have been termed *agnosia*, those of movement *apraxia*. Similarly, there may be *acalculia*, the ability to use number symbols in performing mathematical operations, *agraphia*, the inability to write, and other problems. In any given patient, we may observe various combinations of dysphasic impairments of these types. The various terms describe symbolic deficits; however, they cannot be transposed directly into precise physiological dysfunctions or anatomical lesions.

1 For a more detailed description of varieties of dysphasic behaviors and their terminology, see the references by Van Riper (21), Eisenson (5), and Wepman (23).

Human beings are born with the capacity for learning speech and language, and the correlation of language learning with other stages of development is well known and has been studied extensively. For our present purposes, if we assume a normal developmental potential in the brain at birth, the learning of speech depends on an input from the sense organs and a series of trial-and-error experiments in communication. It is well known that an adequate input system is vital to language acquisition. Children severely isolated from other speaking humans do not develop speech in the usual sense, and deaf children have great limitations in learning to communicate. This learning process requires feedback into the nervous system from sense organs. The child learns to communicate with his parents' symbols, and when he does so successfully he may be said to possess a language, the complex group of symbols used by people of like background for communication with one another and also for the inner organization of their thoughts. The degree to which language develops may be considered a function of intelligence and education. Language and intelligence, though related, are not synonymous. Development of language demands human intelligence, but highly intelligent people may use language poorly. Similarly, loss of speech from a brain disorder does not in and of itself imply loss of intelligence. Both intelligence and language are, however, functions of the brain, and it is not possible to consider one without the other.

This chapter will for the most part ignore the peripheral aspects of speech. By *peripheral* we refer in particular to those more mechanical parts such as the vocal cords, the tongue, the teeth, the muscles of respiration, etc. We are more concerned with the central processes of the brain. The words *aphasia* or *dysphasia* refer to disturbances of speech or language at the highest level of nervous integration. A person may be almost speechless from paralysis of the tongue but not be aphasic. A deaf mute may become aphasic if he loses inner language even though his "speech" had formerly been expressed through sign language. A reading disability is not necessarily due to neurological dysfunction. By dysphasia and aphasia we specifically imply different degrees of the same disorder. The symbols of language and communication are lost or impaired in these disorders and are not the lack of perception of sounds or loss of ability to use and coordinate the muscles to produce them, or bad habits and failure to learn. We thus exclude from our consideration the disorders of articulation, phonation, and primary sensory defects such as deafness or sightlessness, and mental deficiency.

BRAIN MECHANISMS AND LANGUAGE

The central nervous system has developed to its greatest complexity in man. Dominant over all his behavior is the brain with its massive grey covering, the cerebral cortex, containing billions of nerve cells or neurons. The neurons in the cerebral cortex are arranged in layers and are intimately connected with each other in an exceptionally complex but remarkably orderly fashion. They receive messages and work together in mysterious ways so that we may perceive, remember, and think. They operate the muscles, glands, and other effector organs that produce our behavior. Most of the action of the nervous system is unconscious or reflex, and even when it functions as the mind, it brings to consciousness only a small portion of that which is sensed or stored, but in a surprisingly effective manner.

We may conceptualize the nervous system as a hierarchical order, as being composed of a series of levels of functional integration. At the lowest level, the spinal cord with its incoming and outgoing nerves is subject to many and diverse influences descending from higher regions. The contraction of a muscle ultimately results from a nerve impulse leaving the spinal cord by its motor nerve roots. Every movement of our bodies depends not only on such impulses but also on a smoothly coordinated series of influences from successively higher levels of integration. Willed, learned, or purposeful movement, such as the act of writing, thus depends on many levels of the nervous system. Writing requires appropriate motor patterns to move the pen skillfully, but this in itself is only a part of what goes on. We read as we write. We need a check-and-balance system or feedback to monitor the process. Writing even the simplest sentence, therefore, ultimately depends on the highest levels of neural integration, those that subserve both conceptualization and the learned sensorimotor patterns of behavior. It is possible to perform the motor act of writing with no knowledge of its meaning. Anyone could copy a reasonable facsimile of a poem in Sanscrit yet be completely ignorant of the meaning of the symbols used. He could recognize all the visual features of a foreign language and translate these into the fine movements of script but still not know the language. In this book, we are concerned with disorders of symbolic meaning. And it is in understanding these disorders that we have our greatest difficulties in neurophysiology. It must be recognized that we are not yet able to transmute *meanings* into precise physical terms even though we know much about them and although we know how to work with them psychologically. Our experience indicates clearly that the meanings of symbols are related to the functioning of the brain and that speech and language activities have some physical representation in the nervous system.

Much knowledge has been accumulated concerning the relative functional importance of various brain areas with respect to movement and sensation. These are, perhaps, most easily illustrated by abnormalities that appear when parts of the brain are damaged.

2 The reference by Penfield and Roberts (12) will provide the reader with an interesting account of the effects of electrical stimulation of different areas of the cortex on speech and movement.

In general, the left side of the brain has a controlling interest over the right side of the body, and vice versa. Thus, if the entire left cerebral hemisphere were destroyed, there would be paralysis and loss of sensation on the right side of the body, and loss of sight from the right field of vision in both eyes. The individual with such a destructive process, if he is like most of us, would also lose his ability to use speech and language and thus be aphasic.

In discussing the neurology of speech from an anatomical point of view, the cerebral hemispheres assume a major role. As we look at the surface of the brain, it is seen to be divided into two halves that are mirror images of each other. It is dominated by the large cerebral cortex, which can be divided anatomically and functionally into lobes—the frontal, parietal, temporal, and occipital. The surface is infolded by a series of fissures and sulci, which in turn separate the gyri, or convolutions. Buried beneath the cortex are white fibers that form connecting pathways relating one part to another. Also in the deeper regions of the brain there are clusters of nerve cells such as the *basal ganglia,* which are important to posture and movement; the *thalamus,* which in part is a relay station for messages to and from the cerebral cortex and which has as one of its principal functions the distribution of impulses received from the sense organs; and the *hypothalamus,* which is of particular importance in regulating such bodily functions as temperature, metabolism, and the output of water through the kidneys.

Some functional correlations with these anatomical regions can be made with considerable success. It is known, for example, that the area in the frontal lobe just in front of the central fissure is particularly important for movement, whereas the area behind it is vital for sensation. Similarly, the cortex in the occipital lobe receives our visual impressions while the area at the top of the temporal lobe serves as a reception center for sounds.

✓ We must make clear, however, that these delineations are not absolute. We cannot say that a given region is *the* center for a given function. Normal function depends on the working together of many "centers" in a unitary fashion, although some have ascendency over others. The motor cortex appears to be necessary, for example, for the accomplishment of fine finger movements, but playing the piano or typing also depends on a functional inter-

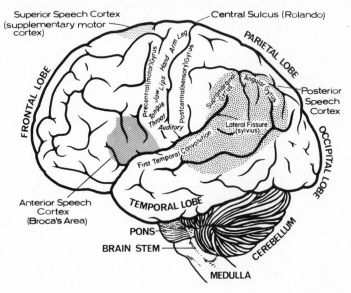

Figure 1. This diagram represents the left cerebral hemisphere of man and demonstrates the major anatomical subdivisions. The right half of the brain has the same appearance in mirror image but in most people a different functional importance with respect to speech.

Areas of particular importance to speech are shaded. The anterior area is of particular importance to the motor or expressive aspects of language; the posterior area with the receptive and formulative functions. The superior area is of less importance and extends beyond the shaded area into the fissure between the two halves of the brain. The diagram of the localizationist might attempt to demonstrate precise areas of the cerebral cortex for individual speech function.

It is to be noted that the anterior speech cortex is contiguous to the motor representation for tongue, jaw, and facial movement in the frontal lobe (precentral gyrus). The posterior speech area, on the other hand, is contiguous with the receptive areas for auditory and visual impulse in the temporal and occipital lobes respectively.

relationship of the motor cortex with many other parts of the nervous system. One of the major problems of the neurologic physician is to be able to localize disease processes in parts of the nervous system, and he uses his accumulated knowledge of functional areas to do so. To him, the combination of various symptoms or physical signs found in a patient may be translated with *great* accuracy to localized disease processes. Thus, an increased briskness of a reflex may signify impairment of the neural pathways coming down from the brain to the spinal cord. Incoordination of movement without loss of sensation and without weakness indicates that the cerebellum or its pathways are affected. Behavioral or psychological testing may similarly yield evidence of focal or areal brain dysfunction. Tumors reflect themselves symptomatically. However, the fact that local brain lesions may be predictably associated with certain defects of function has led many writers to excessive and incorrect precision in localizing presumed functional areas and to rigid concepts concerning the neurology of speech and other disturbances.

3   For an example of the localization point of view, see the reference by Nielson (11).

Two concepts appear to be most important in our consideration of the neurologic aspects of aphasia. The first deals with the greater role assumed by one side of the brain in the integration of speech and language (*cerebral dominance*), and the other with the ability of the brain to adjust itself to a variety of adverse circumstances (*plasticity of function*.) By the term cerebral dominance we imply that one side of the brain appears to take precedence over the other in the neural organization of behavior. Thus it is well known that the left hemisphere of the brain has greater importance for language than the right hemisphere in almost all of us. This lateral dominance correlates well but not perfectly with handedness. The overwhelming proportion of us are right-handed, and speech in some way develops and has its major representation in the left side of our brains. We might, for example, suffer a stroke in the right side of our brain, thereby paralyzing the left side of the body, but still retain our ability to speak meaningfully, although some of our sounds might be distorted. Conversely, if the mirror-image stroke had occurred on the left side of the brain, we would lose not only the ability to move the right arm and leg but also become dysphasic. Our language would be impaired. The "right-brained" individual is a fairly rare specimen in the human race; even the left-handed usually have their left cerebral hemispheres dominant for speech, though, as a group, left-handed individuals do not have their cerebral dominance as strongly developed as do those who are right-handed. Let us repeat: Dominance in the right hemisphere is very unusual even in left-handed persons.

A variety of hypotheses have been proposed as to why one hemisphere is the master over language or why most of us are right-handed. Suffice it to say that none of these explanations are proven. Certainly, although minor anatomical asymmetries occur, none explain why they would be associated with one-sided dominance. Furthermore, in certain persons dominance for symbolic function appears to be mixed, that is, certain areas in the right hemisphere seem more crucial in the integration of certain functions, whereas others in the left apparently govern others. Our experience has been that disease in the right cerebral hemisphere, even in right-handed persons, may impair the ability of the patient to relate himself to his environment or the parts of his body to each other even though he retains the ability to use language. One of these peculiar states is termed *anosognosia,* in which the patient may deny or ignore his left side, may be unable to perceive or recognize that he is paralyzed on the left side, or vigorously deny that he is ill at all. In this instance, we could appropriately refer to the right cerebral hemisphere as being dominant for certain functions concerning the body image. Although there is ample evidence that hemispheric dominance is biologically determined as a genetic or inherited trait, the establishment of speech as a function of the dominant hemisphere is to a large extent a learning process. Handedness is not strongly established until the fourth or fifth year of life, and furthermore, speech function is not permanently lost in cases where lesions of the dominant or left cerebral hemisphere occur early in life. This illustrates the concept of *plasticity of function* of the cerebral cortex, at least as it refers to language. There is no single area to which one can ascribe an absolutely predestined function dealing with speech.

In general we know that recovery from dysphasia due to a given brain lesion is partly a function of the age of the individual. Younger persons recover more readily than older ones. Therefore, it seems that other parts of the brain or of the other hemisphere are able to assume the lost functional roles. In these terms, the young brain may be considered more plastic than that of the adult or older person. This does not mean that all parts of the brain are of equal potential but only that the neurologic organization of higher function is more adaptable in the young. A clinical observation may further illustrate this ability of the brain to make functional adaptation. Aphasia is likely to be more severe with a catastrophic or sudden destructive process than with one that progresses gradually over a long period of time. When death takes little bites, one at a time, the organism is not so hurt. Thus, aphasia is more likely to be more severe after a stroke that causes rapid dissolution of function than when it is due to a slowly growing neoplasm (tumor) in the same region of the brain. It is as if the brain were able to accommodate itself to the slow changes, perhaps permitting other parts to take over the function of the part being damaged. The concept of plasticity, or the ability to utilize other parts of the brain, underlies much of the theoretical rationale for speech therapy with aphasics.

CLASSIFICATION

A variety of approaches to classification of aphasia have been made by neurologists and others interested in speech. At one extreme are those who study language and its defects predominantly from a behavioristic or operational sense and who are not concerned primarily with neural function or, at least, with its localizing correlation. At the other pole are those who might be characterized as the extreme localizationists, who attempt to describe loss of function in terms of specific damage to highly selected areas of the brain. We are reminded of the phrenologist to whom a bump is a function. The brain unfortunately does not appear to be as precisely compartmentalized in the cerebral cortex as would be required for a strictly localizationistic approach.

The speech pathologist may be able to typify a variety of aphasic disturbances with considerable accuracy as to which of the components of speech are impaired or are lost, and he can evaluate the disordered functions that remain. It appears most reasonable, even to this neurologist, to classify aphasia in this fashion, that is, as a behavioral syndrome or as a pattern of psychological dysfunctions.

Most patients who are dysphasic have mixed disturbances. Seldom do we discover that only one of the dissected components of language is malfunctioning. The evidence that a given defect or function is related to a precise anatomic area is actually rather weak, and the danger of extreme overinterpretation is usually present in the clinical reports of localizationists. In our opinion, the correlation of clinical information with exact delimitation in the cerebral cortex cannot be made with any precision. Excellent and predictive correlations are possible, however, if we allow ourselves the same elasticity that nature appears to give to the brain. At present it appears unwarranted to continue naming a speech disturbance, a clinical manifestation, for the area of the brain supposedly damaged. There are further serious disadvantages in ascribing a function to an area when the sole reason for doing so is that the function is lost or altered when that area is damaged. In the dysphasic patient it is a more positive approach to characterize the functions that are retained rather than those that are lost.

Many of the world's most distinguished neurologists have studied aphasia and other related symbolic disorders. In the earlier studies particularly, serious attempts were made to diagram language functions on the surface of the brain. Thus there were developed centers for naming, writing, reading, formulation, music, and many other activities. Often, the demarcation of a lesion from which such centers were derived was inexact, and the description of the speech and language disorder left much to be desired. Rarely if ever does a

4   One of the first scientific attempts to assess dysphasia realistically is found in the monograph by Weisenberg and McBride (22). It is still worth reading.

specific language disturbance appear in isolation or in pure form. The first neurologic studies of speech also began at the time when medicine began to discover the functional subdivisions in the nervous system. Form and function were seen to relate to each other. All students of aphasia will have heard of Broca's area and of the expressive type of dysphasia that bears his name. However, even in the original cases described by this great French neurologist, the pathological process has been demonstrated to have included far more than the area of the third frontal convolution. Furthermore, since his time this area of the brain has been surgically removed without producing any permanent aphasic speech disturbance.

With our cautions concerning the weakness of the strict localizationist view in mind, we must agree that three areas of the cortex are of particular importance to speech as a symbolic function. These are the *anterior, posterior,* and *superior* (or supplementary) speech areas. They include portions of the frontal, parietal, parieto-occipital, and temporal-lobe cortex. A destructive process in any of these areas *may* result in the patient becoming dysphasic. Processes involving the more anterior portions of the brain tend to give rise to predominantly motor or expressive defects with relatively adequate preservation of inner speech and comprehension. The patient with this type of disorder may be able to emit a few words or utter emotionally tinged profanity, but at the same time he appears to understand much of what we say to him. In other patients where inner formulation appears to be preserved but the motor patterns are lost, some neurologists would prefer to use the term speech *apraxia*.

Lesions in the more posterior area, with preservation of the more anterior cortex, are more likely to be associated with disturbances of interpretation and formulation. Often there may be no reduction in speech productivity; indeed, the amount of speech may increase, but defects of comprehension, grammar, and syntax are extremely apparent even to the point of meaningless jargon with neologisms.

Generally speaking, the greater the damage to the cortex, the greater the impairment of function. Smaller or more limited lesions are therefore likely to be associated with less complete disturbances. We have had dysphasic patients in whom only a particular kind of language function was disturbed. It might merely manifest itself as a mild defect in naming or a particular difficulty in reading. When the lesion is massive, all language function can disappear.

The supplementary speech area has recently been defined. This is a region at the superior and posterior part of the frontal lobe. Permanent defects in speech rarely result from lesions in this area, although temporary losses and disturbances of function are shown.

It is beyond the scope of this chapter to classify and characterize the aphasias, and it is impossible to present and argue the justification for anatomic subdivisions among the types of speech disturbances in greater detail. For the interested reader, one of the better recent publications is the small book by Penfield and Roberts (*12*). These authors have made excellent use of the opportunity provided by the performance of brain surgery under local anesthesia to study speech function. Areas were surgically removed for treatment of epileptic seizures, thus permitting the lesions to be more rigidly controlled and precise in extent than in nature's usual morbid experiments. They were further able to interfere with the functioning of small areas of the cerebral cortex and to cause or inhibit vocalization by the application of gentle electrical currents. Although they confirmed the importance of subdivisions of the cerebral cortex to speech, their data and conclusions do not support the concept that we all possess precise cortical subdivisions for given behavioral or psychological defects or functions.

5   Current neurologic thought on aphasia and related disorders is also
well presented in the monograph by Lord Brain (2), a distinguished
contemporary neurologist from England.

DISEASE PROCESSES ASSOCIATED WITH APHASIA

As was pointed out previously, aphasia is not a disease, *per se,*
but a functional defect in language resulting from a destructive
or damaging process affecting the brain. As might be expected, a
wide variety of diseases may attack the brain areas important
to speech. It is characteristic, however, that acute processes affect
speech to a greater extent than chronic ones and that the largest
number of dysphasic patients are those who have either (1) suffered
physical trauma or (2) have had cerebral vascular disease. In the
former, we find war wounds due to penetration by missiles, or cases
in which there are indriven fragments of bone, or depressed fractures
that have lacerated and contused cerebral substance. We have ample

6   For a detailed account of traumatic aphasia, see the reference by
Russell and Espir (14).

civilian counterparts of these injuries among those who survive
highway automobile accidents. Our young adult dysphasic patients
come largely from this group.

Nevertheless, the majority of our patients with dysphasia are those
who have had a cerebral vascular disease. A more detailed description of this etiology may therefore be of value. The term *stroke*
implies an event and the residual defect resulting from disease of
the cerebral blood vessels. The term cerebral *thrombosis* means
occlusion of an artery to the brain by a clot and is associated with
atherosclerotic disease of the arteries. *Ischemia* refers to deficient
circulation. Thus the brain or the heart may become ischemic as
the result of vascular narrowing from arteriosclerosis or plugging
with clot. The term infarction is used to denote the process of tissue
destruction or breakdown resulting from blood vessel occlusion.
Thus the brain may suffer from infarction by occlusion of its blood
supply by thrombosis or by arteriosclerosis or from prolonged
ischemia and slowing of blood flow. It may be similarly infarcted or
made ischemic if plugged with a clot formed elsewhere (even in
the foot) and carried to the brain arteries through the blood stream.
This is called a cerebral *embolus.* Most emboli commonly arise in
the heart and constitute a particular complication of rheumatic
heart disease or of myocardial infarction due to coronary thrombosis.

Cerebral hemorrhage, another cause of stroke, on the other hand, is the result of the rupture of a blood vessel and its bleeding into the brain. Cerebral hemorrhage is most frequently seen as a complication of severe hypertension. Most patients with hypertensive hemorrhage in the brain do not survive. Intracranial bleeding may also occur with congenital weakness of the arterial wall, which leads to the formation of *aneurysms.* These swellings or distensions may burst or form arteriovenous malformations in which arteries communicate directly with veins without going through capillaries, so that pressure is reduced.

Arteriosclerosis, with its resulting consequence, the stroke, is more likely to occur in older persons and in those with special predisposing diseases such as diabetes. Ischemic strokes may be massive or may be small, depending on the site of vessel occlusion and on the ability of other blood vessels to supply collateral circulation. Of particular interest are transient ischemic attacks, in which there may be fleeting episodes of neurologic dysfunction. These episodes of transient aphasia or hemiparesis may therefore forewarn a more catastrophic event. Such attacks may be associated with arteriosclerotic *plaques* (deposits of fat) in the large carotid arteries of the neck that supply the necessary blood to the brain.

As indicated above, cerebral hemorrhage is frequently fatal. Typically the onset is associated with severe headache and a progressively deepening coma. The ischemic stroke, conversely, is more likely to occur when sleeping or at rest, and unless massive or in a particular deep location, loss of consciousness or death will not occur. The brain is particularly sensitive to changes in circulation and oxygen, and the cerebral cortex is permanently damaged if deprived of its blood supply for four minutes or less.

Brain tumors, abscesses, or epilepsy may involve the areas of the brain important to speech and thus be associated with aphasia. Tumors may be malignant (cancerous) or benign. Malignant tumors may spread from other primary sites such as the lung (metastatic) or be primary within the substance and infiltrate through it. Removal of malignant tumors necessitates removal of brain tissue, and if aphasia is one of the resulting symptoms it is likely to remain a more permanent problem. Benign tumors, on the other hand, are more likely to compress the brain from the outside, and if removed, the brain tissue may not be destroyed. Cerebral abscesses have frequently occurred in the temporal lobe, spreading there from infected ears. Focal epilepsy, if involving speech areas of the brain, may also cause aphasia. Usually this will be transient and associated with other manifestations of the seizure. Transient attacks of aphasia and other neurologic disturbances are occasionally seen in migraine.

SOME FACTORS THAT INFLUENCE RECOVERY FROM APHASIA

As mentioned earlier, the age of the patient is an important factor in predicting recovery from aphasia, due in part at least to the ability of the remaining brain to assume new functional roles. This is particularly striking in infants who sustain left hemisphere lesions but who may develop speech at normal or near normal ages. Conversely, aphasia is more likely to be permanent when the locally destructive processes are in older individuals. The reasons for this are incompletely understood as are the ultimate brain mechanisms for any form of learning.

We know that certain areas of the brain, particularly the temporal lobes and the phylogenetically older portions of the brain covered by them, are of particular importance to memory. The mechanisms by which memories are stored in the brain are not understood, and it has been only in the past several years that they have even been approached scientifically. Memory and speech, in some mysterious way, may be chemically encoded in the structure of large molecules within nervous tissue, and those mechanisms with which we "remember" seem to be in the cerebral cortex. Those memories that are more recently acquired are less firmly held by the brain. It would appear that the neural representation of long-term habit patterns may be difficult to change within the brain, another illustration of plasticity or the lack of it as conditioned by use and learning. Loss of recent memory is one of the hallmarks of organic brain syndromes including senility, and the higher-order speech functions are more easily lost in the dysphasic person than are the lower order ones. Primitive aspects of speech may be preserved even in the severely aphasic subject. It is not unusual to see a patient able to emit a few emotionally tinged swear words with anger, pain, or frustration, yet to have no other useful speech at his command.

Other than age, the most important factor is the extent of brain damage itself and, of course, the extent to which the areas important to speech are involved. Brain tissue differs in two very important features from most other tissues of the body. Brain cells do not regenerate. We are thus born with a full complement. Brain cells also demand a continuous supply of oxygen and glucose in the blood and cease to function normally if deprived of either for only a few seconds. The function of a destroyed cell cannot return, but functional readjustment may take place in those that remain. An acute process such as brain infarction in a stroke does not of necessity destroy all the tissue that is damaged or is temporarily without function. In a stroke, symptoms are most severe near the time of onset, and there is a natural tendency toward improvement or healing. We must remember however that an area completely deprived of its blood supply dies. Surrounding this there may be a marginal zone where affected cells live and can recover. In this zone there may be swelling and ischemia but not cell death. Functional recovery is in part associated with healing in this marginal zone. In a given patient it may be weeks or months before one may assume that maximal natural healing has occurred. In a given cerebral insult, one may always hope that there has been minimal permanent destruction. Function may be temporarily interrupted by ischemia, which does not last long enough or is not severe enough to cause permanent structural changes.

Recovery from an acute brain lesion is also affected by the acute functional disorganization that occurs, as will be described later in this text. With a favorable environment and dedicated help, restitution and reorganization of function may proceed on an orderly and predictable course. Neurologists may use the term diaschisis to describe a part of the process of "spontaneous recovery." By this we imply that the functions of connected areas of the brain are altered when an acute process affects one part of the connection. Let us say that parts A and B are closely interconnected functionally by nervous pathways. If part A is suddenly damaged, both parts A and B may be functionless, but with the passage of time part B recovers and even though not able to do all the work of A and B, the total functioning of the patient will improve. These combined phenomena are well illustrated in the sequence of events after stroke with *hemiplegia* (paralysis of one side of the body). If we assume a stroke of major proportions, the entire side of the body may be paralyzed and be without tonus or reflexes (flaccidity). Within a short period of time, tonus returns to flexor muscles of fingers, and then over a period of weeks spasticity develops with associated increased muscle tonus and reflexes. Voluntary movement is more likely to return in the proximal muscles such as the arm or wrist even though the fine movements of the fingers remain affected.

Maximal anatomic recovery usually takes place in the first three months after an acute injury, but there is evidence that healing may continue for as long as a year or more. We can use this information to apply certain rules of thumb to the outlook for recovery for any patient regardless of the type of injury sustained. The longer time away from the injury, the less likelihood there is for recovery on a purely physical basis. Residuals persisting beyond the third month after an acute episode are likely to be those to which the patient must adapt for the rest of his life. Most of subsequent recovery is based on relearning, developing new skills, and adaptation or working around the residual emotional handicap. Rehabilitation can be most successful, but it is not "healing" in the medical context of the term.

The degree to which dominance in one hemisphere is already established in the patient may also be an important determining and prognostic feature in recovery from aphasia. As stated previously, the overwhelming proportion of civilized people have their speech controls predominantly developed in the left cerebral hemisphere. This appears to vary considerably, however, and in some patients it is less well established than in others. This appears to be particularly true for left-handed individuals who usually have the left hemisphere dominant for speech but who may also have a greater tendency toward bilaterality of function. As a generalization we can state that left-handed patients have a better prognosis for recovery from aphasia and will be less severely affected by a given lesion.

7   For another discussion of prognosis in aphasia, see the reference by Eisenson (7).

The factors discussed above seem to be the major *physical* factors influencing recovery from aphasia. To summarize, the prognosis depends on these physical factors: (1) the location nature and extent of the disease process; (2) the degree of "healing" that can occur; (3) the age of the patient; (4) the acuteness of the disease; and (5) the strength of the patient's cerebral dominance.

So far as rehabilitation is concerned, however, we cannot distinguish purely organic or structural factors from those that might be broadly considered as psychological or social. Such a separation is both hazardous and unwise for functional recovery, which is affected by a wide variety of influences. It is equally restricting and unwise to consider recovery of large amounts of language facility as equivalent to complete recovery. It is of course possible that the patient may be able to readapt himself to life and society. The senior author of this text has emphasized these aspects and has himself been profoundly dysphasic but able to continue to make productive contributions to society in spite of it. The person who suddenly becomes aphasic has suffered a catastrophic event, one of great personal devastation and frustration. Any program designed to promote recovery must therefore be directed toward the patient and not solely to the symptoms from which he suffers. For the patient with residual defects, we might aptly describe our realistic goals to be recovery *with* aphasia instead of recovery *from* aphasia. The total milieu is basic to recovery. This includes the patient, the physician, the therapist, the family, the nurse, the employer, and others in society. All may influence recovery either negatively or positively. Motivation is difficult to measure, frustration easy to experience, and rejection is all too frequently the usual response of others when they meet a dysphasic person. The speech pathologist or speech therapist and all others dealing with such a patient must have as their primary goal the aiding of adaptation and adjustment. Rehabilitation for the dysphasic cannot be expressed purely as the return of the ability to use words. It should be of greater concern for us in the health professions to ask what the aphasic *can* do rather than what he cannot. Our efforts in treatment, whether they be called neurological, medical or psychological, should strengthen the strengths that remain, not amplify by our concern the weaknesses that are all too easily seen.

MOST OF US, AT ONE TIME OR ANOTHER IN THE COURSE OF OUR LIVES, experience personal, social, or health traumas. Few of us run the gauntlet unscathed. Some of us fall prostrate under the blows; some of us survive. Ours is a society complicated by many hazards. To endure the vicissitudes that lie in wait for us is no small achievement. To master them is to triumph.

Why do some of us succeed and others fail? It seems quite apparent that the crucial factor lies somewhere in the area of personal security and social adequacy. And these, in turn, seem to rest on the stability of that most important base of the social pyramid, the family constellation. The determinants of our ability to survive and to triumph are often located in the interpersonal relationships of the basic social groups to which we belong. In this book about dysphasia

2   *the patient and his family*

we present a discussion of one of the most severe of all insults to the integrity of the individual. We shall return again and again to the theme that interpersonal relationships are of the most vital importance in determining whether that person will remain hurt or become improved.

Fortunately, man has been endowed with a luxurious nervous system. In adaptability he is outstandingly superior in this capacity —above all other forms of animal life. The human being has proved himself able to survive and to support himself in a fantastic number of different and even hostile environments: in the desert, in the polar snows, in our teeming cities. In recent years he has even demonstrated that he is able to cope with the emptiness of outer space. More incredible is the fact that man has learned to live with others of his own kind and with himself, though in this respect we must admit that his performance has been far from brilliant. It is because man is able to combine facility in communication with appropriate changes in behavior that he has become so creatively adaptable.

Even our cortically traumatized citizens with dysphasia devise ways and means to alter the depths of their despairing loss of function. But their successes are outstandingly dependent on the immediate society in which they survive. Each individual is an entity unto himself and his family. His past is as important as his present, and most assuredly his future will be closely interrelated with both. We must continuously bear in mind that no two persons are identical; the complexity of neurological pathways prohibit such a situation and social histories also make it impossible. To help a person with dysphasia we must understand not only the patient before us but his past and present relationships as well.

Cerebrovascular diseases contribute to a multitude of behavioral, neurological, and physiological deviations. Neurological accidents may result in paralytic strokes, fleeting spells of paralysis, or numbness, gait disturbances, visual disorders, confusion, loss of memory, each accompanied by various degrees of behavioral disruption. The stroke stands in third place as a cause of death in the United States, following heart disease and cancer.

In most instances, until recent years, this tragedy has stripped the patient of all human dignity. At the current time, such patients are receiving clinical care of the highest order with increasing opportunities to reacquire lost functions. Carefully planned assistance eventually restores them to higher levels of personal independence than has heretofore been possible. Though a vast number of patients are quite elderly, significant numbers are stricken while in their early thirties, as they approach the peak of their social and mental capabilities. We must continue to engage in research activities among all interrelated professions and thus establish better and more global methods of rehabilitation.

We wish to stress this truth: brain-damaged adults cannot afford unnecessary social isolation. They retain and regain their verbal facility and functioning only through relatively constant stimulation and through participation in pleasurable communicative experiences within the confines of their homes. This type of personal activity is far more valuable than any regulated remedial drills in our clinics, particularly during the initial stages of the drastic adjustments that must take place.

If we are not excessively anxious to obtain immediate responses from these patients, our assistance is far more likely to result in positive and lasting progress. By patiently and courteously allowing the patients sufficient time to organize their thoughts for verbalization, we often observe that they have far more language ability than the case histories indicate is possible. When such persons are subjected to a continuous barrage of unreasonable speaking demands, however, they may have no choice but to voluntarily abandon verbalization or even completely withdraw from social interaction. If this withdrawal occurs, the resulting depression may result in utter defeat, no matter how many therapists or physicians try to help.

The personnel in every profession concerned with the dysphasic should be exceptionally cautious in all clinical staffings and conferences in which the patient is present. Negative attitudes are terribly contagious. We must always remember that these patients already have more than they can tolerate without hearing the often morbid discussions of the professional staff. There is always present a tendency to forget that the dysphasic has ears and a mind. True, the vocabulary may possibly be beyond the understanding of the majority of patients; but, facial expressions and gestures can be very meaningful to an acutely depressed patient. We must remember also that as time progresses, the patient is likely to have a very accurate recall of nearly all past events. When this occurs, he can lose all motivation for self-improvement and social recovery. We must be acutely aware of the fact that recovery from any illness is markedly dependent on the attitudes of the patients as well as their families. Recovery is also dependent on the attitudes of the attending physicians and therapists.

During the initial phase of the senior author's vascular accident, ten years ago, he asked his wife to keep a daily log of behavioral and lingual aberrations. It is extremely interesting to note that within a two-year period, he could accurately recall *all* major events and conversations without prompting or any assistance from anyone. In many instances such recall deterred his efforts to make social and physical adjustments. One of the most detrimental of such memories concerned the staff discussions of his condition carried on in his presence, even during the first week of hospitalization. Even now some of those comments still come to mind, despite efforts to abandon them. His wife did her utmost to interrupt and prevent such comments and discussions by the visitors who came to see him, but it was very difficult. Even she, a strong, intelligent woman, was traumatized by many of the remarks and speculations because of the possible effect that they might have on her husband's morale. It seems so hard for so many to understand that a stroke is actually a family illness. In any truly effective rehabilitation program, continuous counseling should be readily available for the entire household. Its members should be given an opportunity for frequent contacts with professional personnel since the exchange of both familial and clinical information is imperative. As therapists, the better we know the members of the family the more adept we become in providing realistic guidance for the stricken patient.

Most dysphasic patients cannot overcome their troubles, problems, and maladjustments in isolation. Their homes are often the only world that they will see for many months. Our first therapeutic target must be the home. We must start with the family and help each person in it to see the person behind the patient's chaotic screen of over-all reductions. Since progress is often totally dependent on the factual insights of the persons surrounding the client, we must get the appropriate assistance that will help us solve the inter-related problems that exist in the family group of our patient. Until relative stability, insight, and *appropriate* affection is instituted, there is little any therapist can do to help the recovery of useful language function.

Thus our point of view is that the major need is for guidance, stimulation, and, above all, kind support and reassurance. It is only when these are available that we are in a position to aid the recall and reception of language or its production. For the most part, printed and written words mean nothing unless the patient has a real need for them. Our first task is to create that need.

Despite all the research, we have no truly adequate methods for *accurately* measuring receptive abilities in the dysphasic; they are hidden from our view, but with time and understanding they may emerge. All persons must therefore treat the patient with the same courtesy and consideration as they would have used had the damage not occurred. They should assume that he understands more than he seems to. Even though it appears that he has forgotten or lost a considerable amount of language function, it may be only a tempo-rary shadow hovering over the picture. Our first need is to help him to recall his old behavior patterns and to recognize his place and role in some part of his former world. The family provides this basic focus for rehabilitation.

Dysphasic patients must always be given opportunities and en-couragement to regain physical activities as soon as allowable. We must maintain our contacts with their attending physicians so that we will know how much they can or cannot do. It must be empha-sized that we should allow and accept recurrent periods of emotional ventilation of both the patient and his family. There will be many failures and frustrations, and if there is no one to listen or observe, the patient has no alternative but to drop down into the deepest stages of depression. The dysphasic's greatest enemy is depression.

In the long run, depression can retard or spoil even the slightest recovery of function. Even though the patient is unable to communicate, we and the family should always be available to help interpret and accept the feelings we observe and to provide support in the black hours.

The ensuing chapters will contain but few references to periodical publications. Most research reports are based on means and standard deviations, and the consequent summary discussions tend to be concentrated solely on the interpretation of mean scores. Are we not also concerned with those patients who fall within the deviations from the mean? As stated heretofore, each patient is an entity with a history as well as a geography. For this reason, if none other, it is recommended that you postpone your research readings until after you are thoroughly acquainted with the wide range of individual variations in dysphasia and how it feels to possess it. Research recommendations can then be applied on an individual basis and in terms of the specific needs of each patient. These patients are people, each with an identity and with problems of his own. It is the responsibility of all therapists to provide records of their observations and interactions so that the necessary understandings can be made available to others who may help this person. Each of us must do his utmost to share the unique information our clinical experience has given us with all our other colleagues.

In this we must discard our assumptions of interprofessional barriers. If we are as honest as we wish fellow workers to be, the confession of our clinical difficulties to our coworkers may lead to solutions. Such positive behavior is contagious, and once we are willing to openly admit our own limitations others will do so too. This is not to say that we should be content with our ignorance. There is much for all of us to learn about dysphasia. To cite but one example we should feel obligated to acquire a knowledge of the meanings of neurological terms and medical expressions, if we desire respect and cooperation from medical personnel. At the same time we should remember that an ability to understand or use the professional language of a physician does not mean that we can assume his role or competence. Social murder is unforgivable and it can be just that if any clinician strays too far from his own professional field. True competence is easily recognized and the source of that competence is understanding. This little book is an effort to provide some of that understanding. ᘐᘐᘐ

AS YOU BECOME INCREASINGLY FATIGUED TOWARD THE END OF A DAY that has been exceptionally laden with social and intellectual obligations, you tend to have a higher threshhold of irritability. Furthermore, you often resist even the simplest activity that interrupts withdrawal from relatively unimportant socialization.

Most of you have had broken bones, severe colds with a temporary reduction in hearing, virus infections that produced extremely high temperature readings, or perhaps very simple but painful attacks of gastritis, each of which interfered with social and professional activities. Any one of the disruptions probably contributed to a lessening of alertness and social interaction. How easily have you been able to regulate reactions to just one of the preceding difficulties? It is quite likely that your modifications in personal activities were highly cor-

3 *the chaos of existence*

related not only with the length of time for recovery but with the levels of insight that your family, friends, and even employers maintained throughout the period of your illness. It must be emphasized that each illness probably existed only for a short time and did not impose any lasting reductions in activities. Furthermore, the members of your family group were not overdistraught, which assisted in your retention of a reasonable effectiveness.

Our brain-damaged patient is not as fortunate, for he faces an extremely long period of both personal and interpersonal laxity. Prior to any abstract clinical assistance for communication improvements, we must understand the behavioral deviations that likely result from any damage to the brain. It seems most humane to first consider our patient's emotional reactions. He cannot avoid some feeling of guilt. In observing tensions of the immediate family, the patient is apt to sense that he has altered many living patterns of the persons for whom he has the highest regard. This basic concern, in combination with the multitude of personal reductions, very often results in a persistent desire for complete social withdrawal.

In this chapter we will carefully consider the patient's unpredictable attacks of severe fatigue despite unlimited opportunities for extensive rest. This, if nothing else, lessens the patient's memory span. Another common disorder is that of weakened intellect accompanied by exaggerated elation or depression. Instability is highly correlated with disturbances in visual acuity and auditory sensitivity, both of which may be difficult to detect through isolated neurological evaluations. When such changes are combined with an uninformed household, let alone professional personnel who fail to consider anything other than language acquisition, there is but little chance for the patient to have even the slightest interest in living.

BASIC LIVING NEEDS

At the very least, there are three minimum essentials for positive survival in modern day society. The stricken patient is in particular need of: (1) adequate physiological rest to assist in the maintenance of a more nearly normal psychological adjustment; (2) appropriate nutrition; and (3) the re-establishment of acceptable toiletry. Through the first several months of readjustment, we must remember that these three basic functions dominate attitudes of self-concern.

Far too often, those who have no observable symptoms of body malfunction find it impossible to acquire either a family or professional "ear" to hear anxious discussions of self-concern. When given an opportunity, even "mildly impaired" persons often describe difficulties surprisingly similar to those among patients who are completely paralyzed and have no meaningful use of language. Even though there is but a slight degree of observable neurological damage, such a patient is apt to have a reduction of motor and sensory controls. This assuredly contributes to the negative exaggeration of an organically damaged psyche. Each of us, in the varied professions, too often err in drawing conclusions predominantly based on abstract textbook opinions prior to careful re-examinations, or even casual observations. Clients who are not afforded strong evidence that we are truly concerned may find it impossible to avoid the negative emotional pathway leading to curtailment in behavioral adjustments.

It seems imperative to recall our own reactions to our family, friends, and colleagues as they idly respond to our sincere complaints of health deviations. We have subconsciously been conditioned to make "polite" inquiries about the health of our friends but rarely consider the answer. You may respond to such an inquiry by telling your colleague that you have a severe headache. He may nonchalantly state, "Gee, that's too bad. Maybe you need an aspirin. Oh, by the way, will you finish that report on Jones before you go home tonight?" Immediately you repeat that you just don't feel up to par and may not get it done, but your colleague keeps moving on and has no particular impression of how you truly feel at the moment. Consequently, your headache increases, due to both the tension of working pressures and the apparent lack of sincere concern for your well-being. When *you* are upset by your friend's apparent lack of concern, you are quite likely experiencing a demoralization similar to that which the stricken patient *continuously* encounters.

Fatigue

When we are tired, many changes occur within our own intellectual abilities. Despite any positive motivation you may have while reading this treatise, when you become tired you subconsciously begin to scan these words without absorbing pertinent information. It will become necessary to withdraw from further reading, to seek restful relief and acquire sufficient recovery to interpret meaningfully these printed "squiggles." Your neurological system is capable of making relatively rapid adjustments in the absence of self-imposed pressures. Upon returning to these pages you will quite likely re-establish your reading activity on the exact page, or even paragraph, because you have an ability to retain an abstract level of prefatigue activity. Furthermore, any depressive overlay that accompanied your tiredness tends to disappear quickly and automatically.

Remember, the majority of dysphasic patients have but little vitality, combined with lasting reductions in emotional and intellectual self-controls. Even though our clients may have had enough physical rest to remain awake, they are still far below their pretraumatic energy levels. Lack of energy, of course, contributes to an obvious mitigation in feelings of well-being. Even the slightest degree of excessive pressure may precipitate an immediate return to uncontrollable exhaustion. These people tire easily and tire terribly. With excessive fatigue they cannot benefit from any type of clinical pressure, and even recently acquired physical controls disintegrate. When the patient is pushed unduly, particularly during attacks of fatigue, what has been accomplished may be completely erased, and in some instances, permanently.

Recall your own experiences with high fevers, over-indulgence in studying for final examinations, or the Monday morning inefficiencies following a homecoming football weekend. If one is extremely tired, who cares about polite socializations, let alone the necessity for studying abstract course assignments in statistics, foreign language, or speech pathology? It is true that you must often complete study assignments during excessive fatigue, but you rarely retain sufficient information, despite the heavy threat of examination sequelae. Even your most effective professors lecture badly when they have been under heavy stress or have poor health. If these kinds of behavior occur among those of you who have a physiological ability to return quickly to normality, how much more severely is the alertness of our brain-damaged patient affected?

Neurologically traumatized individuals rarely return to their pretraumatic levels of intellectual and physiological behavior. Attacks of lassitude seem to be unpredictable, for the most part, and variations in their alertness occur far more frequently than those experienced by you. Since unpredictable periods of excessive fatigue persist even among the patients who have lived six to ten years beyond their initial trauma, we should readily expect to find severe and frequent attacks among those whom we contact shortly after their degenerative episode. Chronic tiredness expands reductions of intellectual productivity, memory span, language recovery, recall of immediate or prolonged activities, and the ability to predict future events. All this, combined with the emotional disruptions of their families, can be extremely demoralizing. We must not concentrate on the language disability alone. One of our major clinical shortcomings is the tendency to consider solely the patient's communication deficit with little, if any, concern for the basic attacks of neurological weakness.

Intellectual and emotional responses seem to lack a middle road of normality. Many patients behave in an "either-or" manner, with either extreme elation or extreme depressive withdrawal, both of which are correlated with sudden states of neurological fatigue. There are occasions, though relatively few during the first several months after the initial assault, when during periods of elation they are better able to tolerate abstract levels of socialization. Avoid erroneous reactions to this behavior. It may not be "silliness"; the persons may just feel better. Don't lose valuable opportunities for positive language stimulation.

The majority of our clients appear to be feeling better during the morning hours. A vast number rarely arise prior to 8:30 or 9:00 A.M. It usually takes some 45 minutes to clothe themselves and complete their morning toiletries. Then additional time must be taken for breakfast, which means that the average patient is ready to depart from home around 10:30 A.M. We should do our utmost to comply with the patient's established routine of rest. Unless there is a consistent change in this daily time schedule at home, avoid interrupting routine living patterns for clinical training.

Physical treatments are frequently administered in coordination with our own clinical procedures, and such activities increase over-all tiredness. Avoid scheduling intellectual stimulation immediately following physical therapy. There are very few persons who depart from muscle training without a tremendous fatigue. When they are tired, abstract language sessions are rarely beneficial and contribute only to emotional deterioration. Remember, with fatigue, failures are enhanced and repetitive failures increase the severity of psychological depressions. These may erase any positive attitude toward abstract recovery.

To elaborate this discussion further, we must carefully consider persistent variations in intellectual levels. A substantial number of differences in test scores appear to be highly correlated with a temporary lack of energy. The following case description may clarify absolute necessity for careful interprofessional collaboration:

Mr. W. had wide variations of language usage from time to time and it appeared essential to administer repetitive intellectual examinations to assist in establishing beneficial clinical procedures. Identical intellectual tests were given repeatedly for a ten-day period. Mr. W.'s wife was also contacted for her daily observations of the patient's condition at home.

The vast majority of test results during the morning hours were superior to those in the mid and late afternoon clinic sessions. Early afternoon test scores that immediately followed a two-hour bed rest were significantly better than those obtained during the late afternoon. Even though an identical test was utilized, three times each day, there were consistent and significant differences in test scores. The results of morning testing averaged a score of 96. Following a two-hour bed rest in the early afternoon, test results had an average score of 67. The late afternoon tests, administered with no bed rest between appointments, had an average result of 57.

During this ten-day period the patient did not receive any type of clinical assistance, that is, language training, physical therapy, or occupational therapy sessions. Following an interprofessional consultation, it was determined that each clinic contact should be initiated by the speech pathologist, followed by physical and occupational therapy sessions respectively.

At the end of 30 days, another interprofessional consultation was held, and it was determined that there was little if any observable

improvement. The neurologist noted negative alterations in motor
and sensory responses throughout the afflicted side of the body. The
patient's wife reported a lessening of his emotional stability combined with increased fatigue and consequent social withdrawal. It
was unanimously concluded that the patient had been subjected to
an overabundance of clinical stress. Furthermore, during this time,
his wife's anxiety increased and it seemed to lessen her usual patience
and understanding. All in all, since it was quite apparent that there
was a deterioration in the total family adjustment, formal language
therapy was withdrawn. Regular counseling sessions were initiated to
aid the patient's wife. When a definite improvement in the wife's
adjustment was observed, she was given suggestions for nondirective
language stimulation. Within the following eight-month period the
patient improved his physical controls and made some real progress
in his lingual and social behavior.

The majority of our dysphasic clients have but a limited ability to
withstand even slight degrees of abstract pressure. Each individual
and his family must be considered separately, however, and when
there is a desire for physical or behavioral assistance provide careful
guidance but never exert undue pressure. The rehabilitative process
is slow, strenuous, uphill travel that becomes easier when a carefully
planned pathway is clear and the journey is not made alone.

Nutrition

A vitally important physiological need, of course, is that of nutrition. Our normal population does not eat too little or too much.
There are times, however, when healthy and alert persons have obvious shifts in their dietary activities. Without doubt, you can recall
variations in your own eating habits. When you are on a vacation,
with no need for a specific time schedule, you have independent freedom in selecting both the extent and the kinds of activities in which
you may participate. It is not uncommon for you to fill in your time
with frequent snacks between your regular meals. Most of the munch-
ing activity is a way of avoiding personal boredom. Following an
annual vacation, it is not unusual to resume active employment with
an increase in body weight. This occurs despite the fact that there
may have been some activities requiring physical exertion. It often
takes several weeks to re-establish normal working and dietary activities. Others of you who have had a very active vacation period
combined with a minimal intake of food have experienced an un-

healthy decrease in your weight. When you did find time to eat, you were too tired to enjoy it and maybe even slightly depressed from physical exhaustion. In any event, remembering your own physical and emotional variations may well assist in establishing some degree of insight concerning the physical condition of your stricken cases.

If we are aware of modifications in our patients' nutritional behavior, it will help us to determine their readiness for intellectual assistance. An extremely limited memory span combined with nutritional disruptions often indicates a lack of ability to tolerate any abstract activity. During the first several months at least, a vast number of patients experience serious limitations in recognizing flight of time as well as an obvious reduction in the recall of basic activities. It is not uncommon for family members to become concerned about the patient's unreasonable demands for food. Within an hour after consuming a full meal, such a patient may emphatically demand another complete meal. Once the internal food pressures are no longer noted by the patient, there seems to be no recall of having eaten earlier. Despite the fact that family members carefully remind him it has been but an hour since he has had a full meal, the patient continues to demand additional food. This kind of behavior is often correlated with one or all of the following deficiencies: (1) an impaired judgment of the sequence of time; (2) a lack of reasonable control over the nutritional drive; or (3) periodic variations in the patient's ability to understand the spoken word and inability to recall that a meal has just been completed.

Over-eating contributes to an obvious increase in fatigue. The increased fatigue often initiates a depressive psychological withdrawal from any kind of activity. Many neurologists advise avoiding foods that may contribute to vascular occlusion. Excessive cholesterol limits the blood flow throughout the brain, reduces cortical improvements, and may even result in death. If a patient is unable to comprehend this danger, he is obviously not ready for concentration on any abstract adjustment.

On the other hand, there are a number of patients who have little if any desire for food. This is often associated with damage to the cortical areas that govern nutritional intake, and these individuals are really too weak to benefit even from simple language stimulation. Many insist on complete isolation. Perhaps they do this to avoid extensive feelings of worthlessness as they observe the activities of others. Isolation, however, increases the deterioration of language control. When there is nothing to distract the patient from his personal inadequacies, one may readily suspect a chronically severe depression. Do not hesitate to solicit psychiatric consultations for these families.

There are a multitude of variations in social maladjustments among the varied patients. Continually keep in mind that we are attempting to provide assistance for *people,* each of whom is experiencing numerous physical and social disruptions. A patient is not solely a dysphasic, who happens to be "Mr. Jones," rather he is "Mr. Jones, a person," who has a multitude of reductions, *one* of which is dysphasia.

Sanitary Care

From birth all of us have been confronted with a conditioning process to maintain both personal and environmental orderliness. Consequently, we have a strong subconscious concern for personal cleanliness. There are varying degrees of perfectionism among our friends and acquaintances. The vast majority, however, can tolerate minimal variations, not only in themselves but also in others. Very few become outstandingly concerned if their hair is not combed perfectly, if shoes are not always shined, or even if the razor blade is dull, leaving a minute stubble in comparison with the clean shave obtained the day before.

Neurologically impaired people appear to be overly concerned about these things. This particular form of rigidity may well explain much of the patient's slowness in behavioral recovery. It is most disturbing for the man to lose his independent shaving ability; no other person is really capable of satisfactorily removing all of his stubble. When the dominant side of the body is damaged, shaving is almost impossible with the sole use of his left hand. Even an electric shaver is difficult to manipulate successfully. He is unable to shift the skin to satisfactorily remove whiskers on his chin and neck. Now, as we ourselves are considering this, it doesn't seem terribly important; but the patient is having far more emotional difficulty than anyone can imagine in the absence of a satisfactory abstract attitude. You males should try this with your nondominant hand, not using your other hand, then multiply your reactions tenfold to help understand how extremely important this may be to the patient. Have you men or women ever tried to comb your hair with only your nondominant hand? It can be an excessively frustrating situation, particularly for the perfectionists in our society. Think also how you feel after the barber or hairdresser has combed your hair. In the first place, it just doesn't feel right, and when you look in the mirror, you are also dissatisfied with it. You may either immediately recomb your hair or tactfully wait until you get home or to work. Now, if you among the "normal" population are so subconsciously compulsive, doesn't it seem possible that the stricken patient may feel the same way? When even a so-called "normal population" finds it excessively difficult to accept deviations gracefully, shouldn't we try to maintain a continuous factual understanding of our patient's negativisms?

Many of us have had severe illnesses that kept us in bed for long periods of time. Those of you fortunate enough to avoid such an experience have had contact with either family members or friends who were totally confined. Do you recall your embarrassment and resistance to the use of a bedpan? If you had such a reaction, even though you seemed to make acceptable adjustments, you may readily understand the patient's opposition to his lack of privacy. Even though the vast majority of dysphasics eventually recover enough to depart from total bed confinement, many remain wholly dependent on others to assist in bathroom activities. This need for lengthy dependence can have a devastating effect on any willingness to depart from the home environment, and it can understandably reduce the desire for visitors.

Fortunately, many people re-acquire sufficient motor control for independent ambulation. When this occurs they are also better able to manage most of their dressing activities. Other difficulties arise, however, if there is a reduction or complete absence of sensory nerve tracts throughout the partially paralyzed musculature. A short memory span interferes with prompt attention to basic physical care. Even though such a patient may have a relatively meaningful language expression, the short memory span often creates many embarrassments. When a patient feels a sudden and vital need to go to the bathroom, extensive concentration is necessary simply to stand up, let alone get a cane, crutch, or walker for balance. Once he is standing, the extreme bladder pressure may be suddenly reduced. When this occurs, in combination with reduced memory, he may not remember why he stood up so he sits down again. Almost immediately bladder pressures again become evident, but then, with consequent muscular and neurological fatigue, he may have a complete loss of urinary control. Does it seem feasible, when this person is unable to remember even why he stood up, to expect any positive or lasting results from formal and abstract language retraining in an hour-long clinic session? Such patients are usually unconcerned about extensive recovery in their communication and rarely benefit from formal clinical procedures. It seems obvious that these basic needs are far more important to the patient, and they should also be to everyone concerned with his over-all welfare.

VISUAL DISRUPTIONS

Be constantly aware of possible disruptions in visual acuity. Such deficits can contribute to an expansion of demoralization. Some patients have exaggerated startle responses when they suddenly detect others approaching them from the paralyzed side of their body. They are often thoroughly upset, and meaningful language interaction can be suddenly lost. When we observe repetitions of startle and confusion we must hasten to provide the patient's physician with a detailed account of the occurrences. Total semivisual blindness appears to be relatively easy to diagnose, but degrees of lesser damage may be most difficult to detect. This is particularly true when the patient cannot tell us what is happening to him.

Even relatively minor degrees of visual disturbance frequently have severe negative effects on adjustment. When there is a paralysis to the right side of the body, there may also be some form of blindness in the right half of the visual field. This does not mean that there is total blindness in the right eye. It means that the right visual field in *both eyes* is reduced. The left visual fields in both eyes retain normality as does the left half of the body. It is quite possible for a patient to experience a complete blindness in the upper right quadrants of the visual field combined with a retention of normal acuity in the lower right quadrants. Another variation is total blindness in the upper right quadrants combined with a partial grayness in the lower right quadrants. In this instance, at least, the patient will observe moving shadows in the lower quadrants of grayness and will therefore have some visual indication of the movement of others about him, provided that he is focusing on a parallel plane. However, should he be concentrating on an object in his lap, he will experience a total blindness in the right field. As you may well understand, when he is looking downward, the upper right quadrants of blindness are expanded, the lower gray quadrants are covered by the lower eyelids and he then has a complete loss of visual contact with any activity to the right side. Repeated startle episodes often result in an attempt to withdraw from any social interaction. The catastrophic impact of these visual deficits must be emphasized strongly.

Perhaps a discussion of my personal experiences in a former place of employment may assist in a better understanding of visual involve-

ments. For a period of approximately two years after my initial attack, I had a total blindness in the upper right quadrants of both
eyes and varying degrees of grayness in the lower quadrants of both
eyes. There was a consequent expansion of physical and personal in-
security, not only in my home, but particularly at work. It was difficult to tolerate the flood of persons moving about the hallways, and
very early after I returned to work I found it imperative to keep my
right hand in my right pocket. Unless I did so, due to the combination of right field blindness and an absence of sensory pathways in
my right side, I was frequently embarrassed to discover that I had
belted a passer-by with my flailing right arm. These experiences
assuredly reduced both my social and professional security.

Many attempts were made to reorganize furniture placement in my
office so that I might have my normal visual field in the direction of
office entry. Unfortunately, both the telephone and the intercommunication equipment between my office and that of the secretary
could not be moved. The only solution then, was to keep the office
door closed so that visitors had to knock. I was immediately con-
demned by some professional colleagues who failed to understand
my major motivation in closing the office door. They interpreted this
as a strong desire to completely withdraw from any social activity.
Regardless of my numerous explanations they did not understand,
and I was repeatedly informed that I must avoid withdrawals, particularly in my place of employment.

Over a lengthy period of time there was a gradual and complete
recovery of the vision in the lower right quadrants. Even though the
upper right visual quadrants are still totally absent, my office door
now remains open during the majority of my working hours. There
is still total blindness to any activity in the right visual field when I
concentrate on my desk work. It took a few years to control the
anxieties, and no one could rush it.

In my home environment it was easier to rearrange the furniture
to lessen depressive startle responses with the sudden appearances of
family members and visitors. When I was seated in a position that
directed my good visual field toward the center of entry and household activity, there was far more desire for socialization and greater
control of irritations and depression. The repositioning of furniture,
however, was not accomplished until I had regained a reasonable
degree of meaningful oral expression and could explain why it was
necessary.

My family would have been saved from an extensive amount of
anxiety had they been given professional counseling in preparation

for my return from the hospital. It is also quite possible that meaningful language expressions might have returned more quickly had I not been so emotionally distraught with the observable discomfort of those around me.

8   It is always useful to read personal accounts of recovery from dysphasia. One that will provide some real insights is that of Hall (8).

It is important to stress that many patients experience similar degrees of visual disturbance, and they too have had extreme difficulty in helping their family members understand this particular problem. Someone has to adjust, and it appears that the patients have no choice but to meet this obligation, particularly when professional persons lack a reasonable understanding of the problem.

DISORDERED SURROUNDINGS

There are numerous reports of the perfectionistic orderliness that seems to accompany even slight cortical damage. Such behavior seems appropriate in patients who have visual disruptions. Keep in mind that many individuals are trying to establish a higher level of security by regulating their surroundings. Even people with no neurological changes are far more effective if they approach their daily professional and personal activities with a reasonable degree of neatness. We must keep in mind that the brain-damaged adult tends to behave in an exaggerated manner, hence the concern for systematic organization may appear excessive. It is also true that abstract intellectual abilities seem to be further diminished when environmental disorder occurs. Many patients will try to align stacks of paper, books, or even the paper clips scattered on the desk before they are willing to concentrate on any interpersonal communication. Eliminate distractions; clean up *before* they arrive.

A majority of the patients seek to retain an immaculate appearance and seem overly concerned about their clothing, hair arrangement, cosmetics, and even their fingernails. This may be an attempt to retain social acceptance. These people are often realistically concerned with their personal competence, so help them, don't condemn their attempts. There is, of course, a wide continuum, and even though the majority may be concerned with orderliness, there are many who are not. This might be a carry-over from prior living habits but is often an indication of a widespread cortical disruption.

Acute disturbances may be observed in the way the patient responds to brilliant colors. It has been noted that a vast number of clinic rooms are highly decorated with brilliantly colored draperies, pictures, wall paints, and even exceptionally bright floor coverings. There may also be a multitude of wall mirrors to further amplify these distractions. Far too often we, as clinical personnel, provide colors that contribute to our own enjoyment and falsely assume that our clients are equally pleased with our tastes. However, there are very few brain-damaged adults who seem able to tolerate any brilliant array without an interruption of their concentration on abstract activities. We recognize this fact in working with brain-damaged children. Surely we can understand that it may also exist in brain-damaged adults.

As we recall the likes and dislikes of our colleagues, regarding decorative schemes in various professional and business establishments, we may more readily understand the frustrations of our patients. This is particularly so when we keep in mind that they are likely experiencing abnormal levels of fatigue. Professional personnel must continuously understand the need for color *simplicity* to assist the patient's basic concentration.

Clinical and home environments can be most attractive when decorated with the solid pastel colors preferred by most brain-damaged patients. This point is illustrated by a case in which the lady of the house had to wait until her recovery was sufficient to direct the redecorating. For a matter of several months, she had emphatically refused to join her family in the living room. It contained an expensive and highly colored oriental carpet, coordinated draperies surrounded by brilliant pictures on the walls, and brightly colored lampshades. The few pastel colors were purely accidental. After regaining sufficient communication abilities, she supervised a redecorative scheme. The living room now has pale pastel colorings on the walls and matching draperies combined with a solid colored beige carpet. She also had the brightly colored pictures removed. It is evident that even her family seems to prefer this new decor. This example, of course, is not an extremely common one, but it assuredly indicates these patients' limited tolerance for bright color distractions. Many of your cases will probably want color modifications at home and appreciate the subdued schemes of an orderly clinical environment.

AUDITORY CHANGES

All patients lack some ability to interpret groups of speech sounds. Keep in mind that there may be a disruption in the eighth nerve function on the paralyzed side of the body. It is not uncommon for many patients to indicate an auditory reduction through difficulty in detecting a source of sound. Again, as discussed in the section on visual acuities, we must be sure that we are communicating with the patient from the undamaged side of the body in attempting to determine if there is a continuous damage in understanding, an actual change in the eighth nerve tract, or both. With any paralysis, it is quite possible that the orifice of the eustachian tube may be totally collapsed. Foreign matter may be trapped in the middle ear and result in a chronic infection. It is difficult to procure accurate hearing measurements among those who are highly disoriented. For these reasons, if none other, our first obligation is to arrange a referral to an otologist, who may be able to prevent an additional hearing impairment.

It is advisable to use audiological techniques that are suitable for the very young child. By using simple testing procedures, we may more accurately assist the patient in circumventing further obstacles to the adjustment pattern. Audiologists should most assuredly be included in all evaluative and retraining procedures. It is imperative to administer auditory rechecks at *least* every six weeks to help in understanding the appropriateness of language responses.

Psychogalvanic testing is quite inadvisable for brain-damaged cases. This type of testing is often unwise even for people with no history of neurological trauma. If we keep in mind that our dysphasic patients are extremely insecure, easily frightened, and also frequently experiencing exaggerated sensory reactions to any stimulus, we may then better understand the reasons for bizarre psychogalvanic graphs.

Many respond accurately to pure-tone testing, but it does not guarantee that the patient will have a corresponding ability to understand speech stimuli. If you get a relatively accurate pure-tone response, avoid erroneous assumptions. Some patients respond to language stimuli with accuracy. The room should be sparsely furnished with no stimuli, such as wall pictures, tape recorders, or even a pure-tone audiometer. The patient must be able to concentrate completely on spoken words coming through the loudspeaker. Speech-reception testing may also contribute to an understanding of limitations in the ability to interpret spoken language.

All testing procedures should be as simple as possible. Restrict the length of time for each session, the extent of language stimulation, and above all be constantly scanning the patient's level of physiological exhaustion. It may take many appointments to complete the entire sequence of an auditory evaluation. Always be careful to avoid lengthy concentration on abstract content. Many times these examinations are markedly enhanced when a close family member is consistently present to provide a higher level of security for the patient.

EPILEPTIC ATTACKS

Epilepsy is often difficult for the physician to detect during the patient's relatively brief stay in the hospital. You, the speech clinician, should be well acquainted with the varied types of epileptic behaviors so that the physician may be informed of your observations. If you can recognize the symptoms, you may do much to help. Even though a specific type of seizure has been diagnosed, the severity among repetitive assaults may be altered. For example, consider the patient with a diagnosis of grand mal epilepsy. This classification, of course, presupposes loss of consciousness, extensive body tensions, and randomized physical gyrations. There are many patients, however, who do not always lose consciousness but have some muscular contractions throughout the body, excessive dizziness, or a sudden increase of language deterioration. When milder attacks occur the patient can be aware to some degree of surrounding activities and may understand conversations between others in his presence. So watch your tongue! As he gradually recovers he is apt to suffer increased psychological disruptions such as exaggerated feelings of worthlessness and depression as he recalls the verbalizations of those about him.

In the absence of medical care, epilepsy can result in death. Be exceedingly careful to maintain a close and *confidential* contact with the patient's physician; he will appreciate your observations. Most importantly, the patient will benefit if the threat of severe or even life-threatening convulsions can be minimized. The cessation of repeated attacks, as you may well understand, will assuredly improve self-attitudes and expand the possibility of language recovery.

Always be aware that there will be variations in the patient's energies. Even though he may be under medication to control epileptic seizures, we can never be absolutely certain that subtle convulsions are not taking place. It is fairly common for some patients, regardless of medication, to experience several obvious seizures per year, and when there is a confirmed diagnosis, it is easier to justify the cancellation of appointments. In a vast number of instances, these patients' objectivity and memory spans are severely diminished for a period of several days after an attack. For the most part, they are aware of reductions, and this may increase the seriousness of accompanying psychological depression. No client needs an additional reminder of worthlessness—be sure he is ready to return for further training.

During the first eight months after my initial neurological trauma, I experienced numerous epileptic attacks that temporarily increased dysphasia, confusion, and depression. Unfortunately, throughout my professional training process, I had not been carefully informed of the sudden behavioral variations that accompany brain damage. I was aware of the major types of epilepsy, grand mal and petit mal, but was not closely acquainted with other types described. Consequently, I really had nothing to report to my family or physician. I was assuming that these less obvious seizures were simply a part of my dysphasic behavior, and therefore I accepted physical and social changes. With each attack, I first experienced flashes of light in the right visual field, developed extreme fatigue, found increased difficulty in conversing, and became increasingly irritable.

Eight months after my initial cerebral assault, I had an exceptionally troubled morning during which there was a continuous problem in vision with an increased difficulty in conversing and understanding. The morning ended with a complete loss of consciousness, a rush trip to the hospital, and confinement to an oxygen tent for many hours thereafter. One of the physicians in attendance, who incidentally was also a close personal friend, informed my wife that for a considerable length of time he seriously doubted my survival. After several days of hospitalization I was discharged with a medication to assist in reducing or eliminating future seizures. Fortunately, the medication was most effective and resulted in a gradual and positive increase of time between seizures. Most of the symptoms of epilepsy had disappeared after two-and-a-half years. It is important to stress here that my family experienced more emotional trauma from these attacks than I did. Fortunately I lost much awareness of my severe attacks and could not recall vividly the events that immediately followed them. For several weeks I was a very happy patient because my levels of abstraction were so reduced that I simply had no reason to worry. After my system absorbed sufficient medication to decrease both the severity and frequency of attacks, my levels of intellectual abstraction were markedly improved and in time the situation was normal again.

As you may deduce, many brain-damaged patients experience epilepsy, but there are far too many undiagnosed instances. Unfortunately, those of us working in the areas of behavioral and language rehabilitation are often inaccurate sources of information for our medical colleagues. We must not discuss our observations with the family before they receive medical confirmation, but we must inform the doctor. We have been trained to provide communication assistance, not medical diagnoses and treatments. Observations of medically related deviations must be confidentially reported solely to the patient's physician.

In summary, let us consider some behavioral deviations that may assist the neurologist in re-evaluating the patient:

(1) Sudden attacks of extreme fatigue.
(2) Frequent demonstrations of spontaneous hyperirritability, sometimes accompanied by self-punishing behavior.
(3) Periodic increases in verbal and behavioral confusion.
(4) Instantaneous disruptions in verbal expression.
(5) Unexplained pains in any part of the body, particularly when these occur in the paralyzed side that has not previously demonstrated a sensory response.
(6) Attacks of extreme stomach upset resulting in vomiting.
(7) Agitated restlessness for no apparent reason.
(8) Excessively severe headaches.
(9) Lightning flashes in the visual field.

The attending neurologist may acquire an electroencephalogram when one or more of these behaviors consistently reoccur. This is a painless and harmless procedure. In many instances hidden epilepsy is detected, and with the help of drugs, the attacks are more easily controlled. Deficiencies in relearning may stem from quiet forms of epilepsy, and many victims have such mild attacks that they are unaware of the devastating disruptions. Erroneous impressions such as "organic neurosis," "gastric migraine," "peptic ulcer," and "behavioral disorders" are often deleted when the physician is given realistic information. There is nothing mysterious about what causes cells to go bad when there is a history of brain damage.

Varied behavior

Memory lapses seem to accompany even slight degrees of trauma to the cortex. Many of you may have fainted at some time or other and may remember being confused during recovery. It is quite likely that you had difficulty in re-establishing adequate visual competency, trouble in understanding the conversation of those in attendance, reductions in effective oral responses, a deficit in recalling events that preceded the unconscious state, a feeling that everyone about you seemed to be talking at once, and confusion in organizing reaction patterns. In essence, you were suffering something resembling a *temporary dysphasia.* Voluntary recall of the activities that followed the fainting also seemed hampered almost to the point of amnesia. As memories of the experience were gradually regained, discussions concerning the behavior may have been understood, but an inability to voluntarily recall the specific circumstances would have persisted. It is also likely that those who have fainted experienced exaggerated emotional reactions either of apathy or hyperirritability. All these reactions also occur in dysphasia.

Many dysphasic patients are unaware of memory difficulties, particularly if they cannot even remember their own thoughts during current conversations. They seem to be living for the moment only and do not recognize clearly their social inadequacies. A number of these persons show no obvious concern about their limited intellectual abilities, and we must remember that as long as this persists the patient is not yet ready for any vigorous retraining activities. Deficiencies in immediate recall of current activities is a *contraindication* of readiness for formal clinical procedures.

Even though a patient may reveal instantaneous and enthusiastic willingness to participate in some remedial program, don't forget that there is apt to be significant limitation in memory. A good session of physical therapy, for example, does not necessarily mean that he will remember specific home assignments after departure from the therapy room. A family member or an attending nurse should accompany the patient during most clinical sessions to assist in the continuation of exercises upon his returning home.

Most physical controls are not extremely abstract, particularly when the patient has an enthusiastic interest, but it may lapse once the patient departs from the clinic. It may be helpful to share again a personal experience. I was, and still am, very fond of my physical therapist and consequently anxious to comply with all activities throughout the therapeutic sessions. For a considerable length of time I was told to practice the exercises several times a day upon returning home. I readily agreed to cooperate but was usually so exhausted after the sessions that my wife had to assist me carefully into the waiting car. Having great insight she kindly avoided any unnecessary pressures for communication. After adjusting to the mobile environment of the car, I often started a conversation. Interestingly enough, however, it was extremely rare for me to remember my conversations with the physical therapist, let alone remember what had been prescribed. Indeed, I was frequently unaware of the fact that I had just participated in such a clinical session.

Usually a day or two passed between visitations to the therapy center, and when I returned the therapist inquired first about my home exercises. I was still too brain-damaged to be dishonest and openly admitted that I had not followed through with the assignments. In due time the physical therapist emphatically reminded me to cooperate if I expected any positive results from clinical visits. This negative experience immediately increased my depressed state and inhibited any voluntary discussion with the therapist. There was also an immediate reduction in cooperation so that eventually the therapist got in touch with my wife. The entire situation was truly a comedy of errors. In the first place, no one had made any particular effort to consult with my wife. Secondly, because I had been able to converse appropriately, though momentarily, the therapist falsely assumed that I was able to retain her assignments. Thirdly, it took an extensive period of time to remotivate any desire for physical improvement. I was depressed. I didn't even care if I moved or not, and this acute negativism also inhibited any improvement in communication and social activities. It must be stressed, at this point, that I was often able both to understand language and to express myself with relative accuracy. How much more severely disrupted is the patient who cannot use language? If he cannot express himself, doesn't it seem obvious that physical and social recovery will be increasingly deterred? It seems apparent, when the memory span is too limited for the retention of instructions even for basic survival, that assignments in abstract language learning are more likely to be ignored. Language facility is necessary of course, but it's far more important to most patients to acquire relative independence from physical care, particularly when those about him cannot understand his distorted or incoherent requests.

When we clinicians have a negative reaction concerning our patient's lack of progress, it is advisable first to consider our own ineptness or complete lack of understanding. The degree of behavioral improvement is highly dependent on the attitudes of persons who repeatedly contact the patient.

Difficulties in Social Adjustment

There are various adjustmental disorders among those who have a neurological problem. Mental deficiency reduces the capacity for acceptable socialization, and it is a common reduction, initially at least among our brain-damaged adults. Therefore, it is imperative that we use clinical procedures within the limits of each person's abstract ability. Most patients are not totally or permanently deficient but often appear to be so during numerous attacks of spasmodic confusion.

Some of the behavioral patterns shown by dysphasics are truly symptoms of an organic psychosis manifested by chronic states of unwavering depression or extremes of unrealistic cheerfulness. Each of these reduces the drive to follow through on productive activities. Some patients seem to lose touch with reality, revealing thoughts contrary to fact. They may even appear to hear and see things that do not exist. When a patient experiences a severe state of depression, any drill on abstract language will only increase negative reaction patterns. At times, all of us experience degrees of anxiety, fearfulness, and mild depression. Fortunately, these feelings are usually temporary, and actually they often assist us in broadening our positive outlook. But our dysphasic clients, without insightful handling, can develop *chronic* states of tension and apprehension. Severe anxiety also contributes to persistent sleeplessness, continuous stomach disruptions, and chronic headaches that retard even minimal recovery in language.

Feelings of anxiety may terminate in a severe state of hysteria. It seems quite evident that our dysphasics should be prone to some attacks of hysteria. Don't carelessly ignore your client's emotional trauma: it can increase a loss in the patient's objectivity.

A variety of *phobias* tend to appear throughout the process of recovery. A cortically traumatized person may suddenly develop a strong fear of closed spaces following extensive periods of confinement within an oxygen tent. It is not unusual for a paralytic individual to resist any increased elevation even within his familiar home environment. If this occurs in the realm of maximal security, it is bound to be even more severe in unfamiliar surroundings. Even a slight threat to minimal security often provokes distracting anxieties. If your clinical facility is situated above the ground floor, be particularly careful to lesson a possible fear of empty spaces surrounding the building and seat the patient with his back to the window. Remember, our clients are continuously threatened by their bodily disabilities and easily upset by any threat to physical security. Even you have varied anxieties in unfamiliar surroundings, but you can readily express your concern and easily modify the threats to your security. You have speech and no paralysis.

Oddly enough, moderate levels of functional anxiety often contribute to positive stabilizations. Many times anxieties help the patient to become realistically cautious. Tensions are often protective and contribute to safety as he walks down a stairway or routinely tests the heat of his coffee before he "gulps" it down. Brain-damaged clients possess some realistic anxieties. They are in the process of re-establishing an appropriately protective self-concern. They assuredly deserve the same kind of warm, supportive, and realistic guidance that we extend to young children as they acquire and habituate apprehensions that enable them to survive in a world full of dangers.

Character Changes

Many individuals in our normal society consistently display a variety of chronic social inadequacies. These malfunctions are too often evaluated unjustly by lay persons who apply such labels as "lack of will power" or "weak strength of character." Consequently, many disturbed individuals are professionally ignored until after their conflicts result in episodes of personal degradation. It is quite possible that the long series of social difficulties could have been reduced or even eliminated if they had been given early guidance during the onset of unacceptable behavior. If those who have no apparent brain damage develop persistent character aberrations, it seems apparent that our neurologically damaged cases will have similar problems. We must bear in mind that a cortical accident makes it difficult to inhibit impulses that otherwise would be resisted. The basic cause for character change is most often due to the organic impairment.

Some professionals suspect that dysphasic patients are malingering or inventing their complaints. The *simulation* of tiredness or illness is very rare. If the patient has symptoms of fatigue, he is most likely experiencing a true organic weakness. These people have much to cope with and limited resources with which to cope. Do not forget that the patient is on the inside looking out—he is likely to interpret your inability to understand the true state of his affairs as an apparent lack of sincere concern. Let's hope it is not so. When this is combined with the patient's awareness of his over-all problem, he often develops an unconcealed panic. This reaction expands his feelings of guilt and further stimulates the desire for complete withdrawal. No person should add any guilt to the patient's negative burdens.

Despondency

Nearly every patient, regardless of the consistent degree of positive recovery, will have attacks of emotional regression. A simple failure to tie a shoe lace, arrange a bow on a dress, express the name of a dear friend, or to recall a pleasurable experience of the day before can initiate a lengthy period of severe despondency. This reaction may result in persistent weeping, self-pity, and complete withdrawal from contact with anyone. Any clinical activity may further exaggerate the patient's self-condemnation. When these episodes occur, we are obligated to understand them and provide appropriate support.

Many times you convert grief into hostile exclamations such as, "Why did this have to happen to me?" "They can't do this to me!" "They are too stupid to really understand!" As your clients begin to improve their language expression they may be unaware of using condemnatory phrases. Such "hostility" may be directed toward friends, neighbors, members of the family, working partners, or even you, the speech clinician. It must be stressed again that most episodes truly represent a denouncement of personal deficiencies.

Unrealistic restriction to a protective environment lessens contact with outside activities such as a former place of employment or even the "old poker club," and interferes with any escape from melancholy. Sometimes it seems as though we should return to the ancient custom of providing black veils or black armbands for displaying a state of mourning. Remember, apathetic professional personnel further exaggerates the patient's loss of positive drive. Watch yourself too.

Final stages of emotional adjustment are usually detected through definite recognitions and acceptance of existing reality. Always bear in mind, however, that this does not necessarily mean a return to the "old self." When a patient begins to feel an increase in emotional stability, he will be apt to expand the variety of his activities. Elevated objectivity contributes to an increased need for communication, and when fatigue and despondency is reduced, there is more hunger for socialization. A word of caution is appropriate here. When positive progress appears, each professional person must meticulously avoid unreasonable pressures. We are to guide, not push patients along the pathway of readjustment. An overabundance of praise tends to completely eradicate the patient's gains; it is extremely difficult to resist any sharp stimulus of excitability. Always remember that feelings of despair are too near the surface. When failures occur, as they always do, the patient is often unable to cope with them without entering the protective walls of isolation. Numerous patients fail to recapture lost gains in adjustment simply because clinicians carelessly exert extensive amounts of pressure for success. The vast majority of improvement comes from consistent but nondirective stimulation and insightful guidance. Positive, nonthreatening, and pleasurable activities help distract patients from a grievous concentration on permanent reductions.

OUR EMOTIONAL STABILITY IS HIGHLY DEPENDENT ON HOW EXTENSIVELY we understand the basic facts of our social survival. Everything about us is continuously changing; nothing is static, particularly our mental and physical health. As clinicians, we are obligated to provide extensive guidance for the families of our dysphasic clients. Far too often these families remain totally isolated from the patient and the agencies that might help them. They are forced to function in terms of erroneous guesses, fears, and unwitting rejections. Professionals must remember that when any clinical evaluation is based solely on a *casual* impression of familial stability, unforgivable blunders can ensue. There can be little hope for brain-damaged clients until we understand fully the attitudes of those around them. This understanding cannot be determined by hearsay or on the basis of casual

4 *familial guidance and education*

or brief consultations. Most families vary in their anxieties and anticipations to an alarming degree, particularly during the first several months following the patient's accident. They are in dire need of warm factual guidance if they are to establish any semblance of stable support for their loved one. It takes considerable time to develop a solid base for the security that means so much for a favorable prognosis.

When dysphasia suddenly invades a family, even the well members of the patient's environment can experience a disturbance in their use of language. Some talk excessively, almost frantically, but make little sense in their state of confused misery. Almost afraid of silence, they seem unable to be quiet. They chatter nonsense. Conversely, others react by becoming dreadfully silent, apparently fearful of verbalizing their concerns. Some retain static facial expressions, such as a continuous but inappropriate smile, a perpetual sadness, or even the undefinable blankness of a mask. You will find most of these people, at either extreme, in need of your help. Both groups are confused; both are overanxious and just cannot communicate either to their own satisfaction or to that of their listeners. Most of the excessively verbal ones have no one who can stop talking long enough to hear them out. The excessively quiet ones may be too demoralized to define their concerns. Many are continuously fearful that they are in part to blame for the patient's illness or for its continuance. Some experience a combination of these erroneous attitudes.

We must persistently keep in mind that the vast majority of these people are reacting much as would most of us should we be confronted with the same trauma to the family unity. Despite our professional objectivity we too would find the adjustment very difficult. Very few of us would be able to view our mates, offspring, or even our closest friends with a strict and nonwavering attitude of problem-solving. For this reason, if none other, we must be cautious to avoid false conclusions or snap judgments about the disrupted behavior of familial groups. Instead we must stimulate them to discuss their personal concerns, hear them out, and help them understand.

Despite good counseling, some members of these families never seem to overcome their silence or meaningless verbal rambling. As a matter of fact, if this rigid behavior persists, it may become worse and further devastate the patient's recovery. Do your utmost to prepare them to shift their attitudes, to create a favorable clinical climate and refer them to those who are qualified to evaluate their emotional states.

PSYCHIATRIC MANIFESTATIONS

The process of adjustment may be better understood if we briefly review the map of major emotional disturbances. Speech clinicians are not trained and do not have sufficient experience to treat profound melancholia, even though all of us have experienced personal but brief attacks of the blues. We must continuously avoid making blind assumptions. Only well-trained personnel in medicine are qualified to undertake the evaluation and treatment of the neurological and resulting psychiatric disorders. We may assist by referring clients when we suspect extreme behavioral deviations, but none of us is qualified even to imply any specific psychiatric disorder. We must clearly understand that these disturbed individuals may have real problems. Wives and husbands of the stricken patients are profoundly shocked by the sudden and extreme changes in their mates.

Prepsychoses

Symptoms of *hysteria* are often noted in family members through various physical complaints that seem to have no organic foundation. For example, as clinical contacts with the husband of one stricken patient progressed, we eventually became aware of his physical discomfort and awkwardness. After numerous inquiries about his health, he finally described cramps in the musculature of his left arm and hand. Knowing that his wife was paralyzed to the left side, it was natural to follow through and ask him how long this condition had existed. Upon learning that the cramps began the day after his wife's embolism it became apparent that he may have developed a functional disorder. An immediate referral was made for neuropsychiatric attention, and shortly thereafter we were informed that he was suffering from hysteria. This readily explained our lack of progress with him throughout the first several weeks of our consultation.

Another type of disorder can be revealed through a constant appearance of fatigue, weariness, sadness, boredom, and resistance to advice or criticism. Such behavior is a symptom of *psychasthenia* and is often overlooked because compulsions, phobias, and obsessions are not readily detectable in our clinics. It seems quite natural that wives or husbands should be sincerely anxious about the condition of their spouses. However, when an apparent obsession about personal survival results in an obvious loss of weight and a nonwavering rigidity of self-concern, we must be alerted. Even though we may anticipate eventual stability, we must make sure of the basic facts and refer such individuals for a medical evaluation immediately. The stricken ones are highly dependent on maximal stability of self-attitudes among other members of the family group, and so are we if we are to help.

Psychoses

We also meet a few individuals in the families of our patients who have had a long-standing behavioral dysfunction. The final blow of their mate's sudden assault can easily expand their instability into a full-scale psychosis. The American Psychiatric Association classifies four main types of functional psychosis: *schizophrenia* (dementia praecox); *paranoia; manic-depressive psychosis;* and *involutional melancholia.*

Individuals suffering with intense *schizophrenia* lack emotional tone and reveal verbal irresponsibility. Numerous negative fantasies explain the tendency toward seclusiveness. They are self-accusatory and sometimes self-glorifying. Schizophrenics are not easy to relate to; their delusions are bizarre, and their daydreaming is more than whimsical imagery. They take their daydreams completely seriously and act as though they are positive facts. Self-centeredness dominates their hallucinatory behavior with little concern for those who love them. They have what may be described as a "perceptual cancer" and once it starts to spread, it does so with alarming speed. Be careful to help slow it down by getting assistance from those who have the deterrents. Dysphasic patients are in enough trouble without having to cope with a mate's loss of sanity.

All of us have experienced brief emotional episodes similar to *paranoia,* wherein the major symptom is that of unrealistic suspicion —the foundation of negativism. It stands to reason that occasionally the wives or husbands of the stricken patients may possibly show strong, but temporary, symptoms of this personality change. When there are *continuous* feelings of such inferiority and guilt, there seems to be no route to any realm of security. Such persons assume that others regard them as they regard themselves, that is, as possessing a fictional sense of worthlessness. Delusions that others are spreading scandalous rumors about them deepen their depressions and continuously expand the base of paranoia. When this occurs, their neurologically impaired mates also tend to exaggerate their own social and physical incompetencies. Persistent paranoia requires comprehensive and highly trained assistance from qualified personnel. You are a language clinician, so get some help to avoid making any blind and disastrous assumptions that create roadblocks in the patient's highway to security. Be realistic and investigate the accuracy of the negative but brilliant statements coming from the wife or husband.

Very few people have escaped either a sense of overelation or attacks of the blues. Fortunately, most of us manage to stabilize our attitudes relatively quickly. *Keep one major point in mind:* normal shifts of mood are hardly sufficient to let you assume that your mild experiences are even relatively similar to those of your extremely disturbed clients. Has anyone ever been as unhappy, worried, or sick as you have been? When you were in a mild and brief state of melancholia have you even cared about the experiences of other people? Did it make any sense when others told you everything was going to be all right? Your answer to each question is quite likely an emphatic "No!" Bear this in mind as you contact family groups.

Manic-depressive psychosis has the peculiar feature of circularity. The behavior pattern is unpredictable and shifts back and forth from extensive depression to unrestrained exultation. Some people may stay exclusively on the depressed level while others must be classified as *manic-depressive-manic.* Those who reveal restricted verbalization may truly be near to or within a classified psychosis. They are despondent within their heavy clouds of remorse. Pessimism, sorrow, and regret reign. They are all but completely drowned in negative evaluational exhaustion. A well-trained lifeguard is essential for such individuals. He will be able to help the family member verbalize the self-sorrow and to relieve the pangs of utter despair. Persons in the manic state are apt to be incredibly comical with incessant randomized verbalization. During a professional internship at a psychiatric hospital, I was impressed with one patient in particular: he seemed to make sense with most of his nonsense. Had I not been aware of his diagnosis it is doubtful that his psychotic behavior would have been detected. Throughout the entire semester he came to the window and shouted, "My sister is unhappy with her baby! His toes and nose look like bows! Ha! Ha! Ha! I'm going home to brace them straight!" Then very quietly (it was several weeks before I understood it) he said, "He's an Indian and can't find an arrow." The quiet portion had a trace of sanity—a rather strong trace. All Indians should have arrows. The speech clinician must learn to listen with strange ears. He must hear *everything* said and give the patient appropriate guidance.

Depression is relatively common during the "change of life." Menopause often creates an outstanding reduction of vitality and hope. It has been suspected that the male is also subject to a similar physiological change, which in itself can be serious enough without further emotional disturbances. A large number of stricken patients and their mates may be going through this maturational process when the trauma of dysphasia occurs. *Involutional melancholia* is likely to show itself in varying degrees of intellectual reduction, memory loss, and general befuddlement. Unreasonable fears and bitterness become increased and often create suicidal tendencies. We must be careful to keep this in mind and seek professional assistance before we delve too deeply into the management of these persons' lingual-emotional behavior.

Suicidal Contemplations

We must also be sure that the family has a clear conception of the dangers of detrimental depression. This is indeed a tender problem for both the patient and those within the household. How does one raise the issue of suicidal tendencies without creating additional anxieties among the family members? How can we ensure that we are lessening the probability of suicidal success?

Most of us have momentarily experienced utter despair together with a serious but fleeting thought of "ending it all." Many of us have been utterly shocked when a close friend, casual acquaintance, or even a well-known public figure terminated his own life. "Why he's always been so jolly." "She has never complained about anything." "He was so successful, alert, and congenial." We must remember that from the day we were born we have been conditioned to appear pleasant, to act joyously, to conceal anxieties, and to avoid expressing negative self-concerns. It is "sinful" to contemplate, let alone bring about our own death. Call it what you wish—sinful, cowardly, or psychotic—suicide occurs, and wishful blindness will not solve the problems of those in hopeless isolation or despair.

Depression among brain-damaged people is not a fleeting or even a casual state of emotional deterioration. It is persistently serious. It is a dominant part of the problem. It takes considerable time to lessen depression and demoralization in these patients, and there is little if any chance for any improvement in abstract behavior such as language and articulation until after the patients are able to perceive some *positive* aspects of reality. Depression retards recovery. These persons are organically confused as well as functionally distraught for a long time after their accidents. Suicide is a constant threat, particularly if we in each profession carelessly ignore our patients' emotionality and weakened familial stability. Let us consider three specific situations:

A middle-aged male, who had been a public school administrator in a heavily populated county, ended his life with a gunshot while his wife was at work. He had recovered sufficiently for independent ambulation some three months following his cerebral embolism. Six weeks after his cerebral accident, he was enrolled in a speech clinic and attended remedial sessions three times weekly until the time of his death, eight months later. He was pleasantly cooperative and had a smile for everyone despite severe attacks of fatigue. *After* his death, his wife was offered supportive counseling by a former colleague of her husband. She refused by stating the door was closed when she needed it the most. Had she been even slightly aware of his demoralization she could have disposed of his hunting gear. She had never been given any detailed guidance, even from the speech clinician.

A young physician, in his early forties, suffered a cerebral hemorrhage. Physical therapy began while he was hospitalized. A speech clinician was contacted when he returned home, and language drills started immediately. The patient was slow in responding to anyone, let alone the therapists and their clinical activities. He showed obvious facial and behavioral symptoms of severe demoralization. A few professional contacts were made with his wife but they were excessively casual, professionally verbose, and far too brief. Approximately one year later, he shuffled into the room that contained his medical supplies and consumed an overdose of barbiturates. He left a sparse but somewhat meaningful note; "Hell (Help?) no gud (good?) Jan (Jane—his wife) Kri (cry?) sari (sorry?) for yu (you?)."

9   An interesting account by a physician of his attempts to regain language mastery is found in the reference by Rose (13).

Lastly, another stricken adult, a university professor with a Ph.D., made some unsuccessful attempts at suicide. He seemed to be unaware of his activities at the time of his episodes. Both times he arose in the middle of the night, turned on the light over the bed, went into the bedrooms of his children and turned the lights on, and also lit up the hallway and the bathroom. He secured a razor blade from the medicine chest, kneeled before the toilet and dropped his paralyzed arm into the water. Although his wife had followed him into the bathroom, he seemed to be totally unaware of her touch or attempts to talk to him. As she was removing the blade from his good hand, he suddenly regained consciousness and questioned the activities of those around him. The second episode occurred in the kitchen, and his wife removed a carving knife from his grasp. Both he and his wife later speculated that the behavior was highly correlated with undue pressures from fellow professors, once occurring during a home visit and a second time after he had been subjected to unreasonable stress by one of his colleagues during a brief visit to his office. Despite the obvious show of suicidal attempts, his wife was never given professional assistance for even this specific emotional distress. Our interprofessional obligations seem obvious. We must remind the family groups to keep destructive medications, firearms, and dangerous utensils out of sight, or better yet, out of reach. Most of all, we must listen to them, talk to them long enough to drain their excessive anxieties before they depart. At an appropriate time we can then bring this possible threat to light. Don't stab them with a dangerous question and immediately run away. Above all, let us remember that clinical training for the patients themselves is obviously detrimental until they have made some recovery of reasonable emotionality.

SEXUAL DISRUPTIONS

In due time, there is bound to be some degree of anxiety regarding sexual relationships of the marital union. Such maladjustments are lavishly discussed in the professional literature of psychiatry and psychology, but the literature dealing with the dysphasic per se is sadly lacking in this particular aspect. There appears to be no reference to the frustrations experienced by the well members of these marital partnerships. True, this is a very personal affair, but so are all problems of adjustment.

A large percentage of your patients' wives or husbands will, if given an opportunity, discuss their sexual concerns about both their stricken mate and themselves. For the most part, an understanding of their patient's change in sexual drives and the probability of adequate recovery is readily effective. However, we should acquire both specific medical information and permission to discuss the matter *before* we initiate any contact with the patient's mate. In this manner we are then prepared to respond immediately whenever the appropriate time arises. The speech clinician must again work closely with the physician. We must also remember that nearly all degrees of personality deviation reveal symptoms of sexual instability and often interfere with the willingness to discuss them.

With an acute understanding of the stricken mate's deficit in emotional concentration and the extreme limitations in memory span, it is often easier for the well mate to understand that a lack of sexual drive does not mean personal rejection. Most patients eventually regain their sex drive, but initially they lack concern for the satisfaction of their partner, and this can repel and produce conflicts. If the well mate can understand that the entire process is very similar to their honeymoon and the early months that followed, that new adjustments must be made, then the current disruption of relationships can be viewed more realistically.

The physical appearance of these patients also tends to eliminate the desire for intimacy. This is particularly so if pretraumatic unions were unsatisfactory. If such conditions had previously existed, a number of other personality traits may have also been distasteful. All these attain undue prominence after the attacks. Often there is little motivation to assist the patient in any respect. The most common form of sexual maladjustment, among the general population, seems to be that of simple prudishness. Shame and fear may have been developed in early childhood because of parental attitudes.

Frigidity and impotence can then be the ultimate consequence following a neurological damage to the marital partner. This particular deviation may, however, be confined only to the husband or wife, and it can expand into a total rejection of the patient. If this occurs, the speech clinician should recognize that the dysphasic may lose motivation for any social recovery or even lack any desire for language recovery.

A number of individuals seek sexual satisfaction with persons other than their stricken mates. In our society this behavior is unacceptable, and promiscuity can readily expand basic insecurities. It is evident that some freedom must be provided for discussion of sexual anxieties. There is little that we can do to help the patient increase verbal competence if underlying tensions of the marriage are not maximally reduced. If we have any doubts we should stop and refer such individuals to a properly trained clinician in medicine, psychology, or marital counseling. A psychopathic personality lacks normal inhibitions, is pervasively immature and unreliable; so get help for him early enough to arrest further deterioration in the beneficial attitudes we need for language recovery.

WHERE SHALL WE START?

By the time the distraught members of the family come to us, they are likely to be fed up with cold factual inquisitions. They want to be considered something other than an entry on a statistical table. If we have made the proper preparation for the contact, the basic medical facts and social summary are already in the clinical folder. If not, simply get the name and address of the attending physician. A vast amount of information will be forthcoming from all the members of the family once they sense congenial freedom for their discussions. Don't be a normal person; be abnormal—listen to them! It is unfortunate, but nearly everyone, professional or not, is so busy advising, orally analyzing, and impressing themselves that they must keep verbalizing even before they know if there is any need for most of it. You may recall that on numerous occasions your own emotional ventilations have been abruptly halted. Your colleagues, friends, and even professors have interrupted to discuss their own personal woes. Very few persons have listened without monopolizing your conversations. Avoid doing this to your clients' families—listen and let them complete their expressions of self-concern. Helpful suggestions are impossible until we know what kind of need exists. If you do not listen, most of your clients will ignore your impertinent ramblings and quickly disappear from sight.

A word of caution! Don't be a poker-faced listener. These clients need observable indications that you are hearing what they say. Their world is already too full of unresponsive fence-posts. How long do any of *us* talk to those around us when they do not take time to listen or when they do listen fail to let it be seen? We need to see that our friends are really interested in our conversations, otherwise there is no need to ramble on. Certainly our patient's family needs no reinforcement of their despair. Hardly anything does as much good as a warm smile, a raised eyebrow, or an interested gleam in the eyes of the listener, a brief verbal reflection of what they have been saying. A good clinician is sincerely interested in hearing them and lets it be seen—if he is bored he should get out! It is not necessary that we be god-like, continuously providing answers to every quandary. People often find their own solutions as they discuss their self-concerns. In an atmosphere of congenial interest this talking-out activity is satisfying, self-corrective, and relieving. In other words, the extent of anxiety seems to be highly dependent on how much these family members can hear themselves think out loud in the presence of sincerely interested professional personnel. When they themselves become aware of their emotional pitfalls, they are more apt to avoid the terrain of hopeless defeat.

Let us take a moment to coin a word that may subconsciously enhance our positive effectiveness with a warm objectivity:

Sempathy: A feeling of sincere warmth and compassion for another's troubles (sympathy), with sufficient emotional control to factually evaluate the needs of others (empathy). An attitude of warm relaxation and reassurance combined with a careful view of existing circumstances.

Remember, the people we see are not abstract statistics; they are warmly concerned, and we have no right to make any false assumptions that they are not. One thing must be made clear at this point. The families we are now considering are not on the borderline of any psychosis. If you listen, they make a great deal of sense with a minimal shadow of nonsense. They are capable of recognizing their expressive repetitions and are in the process of sharing their trauma with a "sempathetic" clinician. After they hear their own thoughts and anxieties there is an improvement in their ability to make better sense. In time, *they* become good listeners, and their questions become more meaningful as we assist them to clarify their inquiries. Keep in mind that most dysphasic patients are a product of their environment and that it must be reasonably stable if they are to re-acquire a satisfactory existence.

Perhaps it would be helpful to regress for a moment and recall the process of language development in younger years. It is quite evident that positive socialization is the major base for the pyramid of communication. However, some youngsters seem to exist in a social vacuum, and for them there is little verbal stimulation let alone reward for language expression. Their "wailing grunts" acquire sufficient attention for sanitation and nutritional needs, but otherwise they are isolated from any verbal interaction. When there is no need for speaking, and when this is combined with a sense of rejection, normal language development is bound to be disrupted. Conversely, overprotection and stifling affection also disrupts the process of language development. There is no need for words when the youngster's slightest groan or laughter acquires immediate and rewarding attention. Our own professional literature and our professional colleagues stress familial change and education to assist in the remedy of initial communication retardation. True, this particular group of children has no apparent neurological deficit. Their future is hopeful if appropriate familial insight can be achieved. This, also, includes relative freedom for interaction with peers outside the home atmosphere.

The majority of emphasis, in the literature dealing with dysphasia, is concerned with the patient's neurological, physiological, and language deficiencies. Discussion of familial guidance is often too casual and is consequently overlooked. These families seem to experience far more trauma than has heretofore been vaguely implied. Ignorance with respect to dysphasia is *not* bliss—it is devastating. The wive's or husband's expectancies are bound to fluctuate from day to day if they must fumble in isolation. Infantile behaviorisms in adult physiology can be intolerable to those within the household, particularly when the latter possess no broad and factual understanding of the disorder or of themselves. We must be, at the very least, as kindly supportive with the families of dysphasics as we are with the parents of young children who have failed to learn to talk.

Ideally, the basic information regarding the multiple aspects of neurophysiological disruptions should be provided by the attending physician prior to the patient's dismissal from the hospital. In this manner, the patient's relatives will be given some cautious anticipation and be more apt to recognize the necessity for regulated contact with medical personnel. It is also advisable to provide them with explanations of behavioral and language problems to be expected and to impress the family with the fact that such deviations are common among these patients. No one likes to feel isolated and no one should be. If at all possible, referral should be made to a competent speech clinician within their community. Those living near one can be quickly enrolled for assistance in one of the local speech clinics. We in speech pathology are obligated to carefully define our role, not only to the family group but assuredly also to the medical personnel concerned. All must thoroughly understand that we recognize our professional boundaries, and should the family have an inquiry about the patient's health, they will be immediately referred to their attending physician for further counseling. We must not play doctor.

VARIED FAMILIAL CONSTELLATIONS

There are many varieties of familial constellations related to the problems of dysphasia, and each requires careful consideration. There are no rigid clinical routines appropriate for each and all, and we must remember to take into account the following variations: (1) The age levels of the patient and his (her) mate; (2) the education and employment backgrounds; (3) the social activities that the patient and mate particularly enjoyed; (4) the mental and physical health of the patient's mate; (5) the emotional attachment between husband, wife, and other members of the family; (6) the ages of the children within the household; (7) the parental adjustments to the youngsters and vice versa; (8) the interchild relationships, and (9) the over-all social drives of the family group. Obviously this is but a partial listing of the numerous variations, but it is essentially a basic core of those most commonly seen. As stated earlier, there is no one approach that will satisfactorily assist *all* families, and this fact alone strongly supports regulated consultations over an *extensive* period of time.

Help for the Elderly

A significant percentage of the dysphasic patients referred to our clinics are beyond the age of retirement. Many have already experienced a progressive decrease in their social activities. Some of their life-long friends have departed from the community, and some are confined to their homes because of chronic physical or mental health problems. Varied degrees of senility have developed among some of their acquaintances; others are deceased. Continuously bear in mind that some of your elderly stroke patients may have been very senile before their accident. This may also be true of their "well" mates; that is, they too may have become senile several years before you came to know them. Be sure that you acquire this information before you initiate extensive counseling procedures. *Organic social death* is no easier to rehabilitate than death itself. Furthermore, when you observe symptoms similar to senility, refer the individual to medical personnel immediately. Many new treatments that can deter the rapidity of degeneration or even prevent the initiation of the devastation are now available. If you carelessly ignore existing needs, it strongly interferes with the patient's desire for any recovery.

Clinical counseling for the aged, of course, is not always an immediately rewarding experience for many reasons. Most assuredly there will be but little benefit from family contacts if the patient has to be left at home in isolation during these sessions. It is most unwise to leave such a person unattended. If it is medically feasible, make arrangements for both patient and mate to come to the clinic. Even though the patient may not be ready for any specific or formalized retraining procedures, he will at least have a different companion who may assist in stimulating a desire for verbalization. His wife will then be in a better frame of mind to discuss her concerns and be more attentive to your professional guidance. When there are monetary limitations, however, it is sometimes impossible for them to manage the transportation from home. Aid may be forthcoming from fraternal lodges, church groups, voluntary societies, governmental commissions, or even interested individuals within the community. A listing of these sources should be appropriately dispersed by our centers. If at all possible (it is if we want it to be), we should make an occasional home visit until transportation is arranged for the aged couple. In this manner we have an opportunity to demonstrate our sincerity, lessen their feelings of hopeless isolation, and very importantly, pick up some cues to enhance our counseling sessions when they come to our clinic.

It is particularly important for us to bear in mind that elderly persons tend to resist directions from the "youngsters" of society. Their attitudes are quite similar to ours, so let us examine our own experiences at home. Even though an eighteen-year-old son has a vast knowledge of the automobile engine—and Dad doesn't—it is often extremely difficult to accept this fact willingly because, "My son is still just a kid." And so it is with the young daughter who is designing clothes—she too may have a hard time convincing Mom that she really knows what she is doing. Many of our aged clients subconsciously feel the same way toward us, the kids of the professional world. If we are careful to avoid immediate and extensive direction, positive results are more apt to be forthcoming. They must feel us out in order to gain confidence in our suggestions. We must reveal our competence.

Occasionally a family member is mainly concerned with her own problems, many of which seem to be totally unrelated to those of her patient. This self-centeredness may have existed long before the current trauma. We cannot deny her need since it is doubtful that she will ever truly understand the plight of her sick mate until her own personal dilemma is reduced. Sometimes the only route to the patient is through an emotionally sick family member.

Even though it is extremely difficult to face objectively, we must also recognize another fact that exists among the elders in our population. The life expectancy of both marital partners is markedly limited, and many of them are acutely aware of this fact. If such people are living almost solely for their mate, the major concern may not be that of regaining useful language. Quite often there is a sole concentration on physical recovery—if they have the strength to follow through. The spouse may not care so much about the recovery of the patient's language as she does about the preservation of his physical presence.

The memory span of the aged patient is apt to have been shortened long before the accident, and satisfactory conversational activities have long been limited. As one may easily recognize, there is not a great deal for them to talk about, nor are there many persons with whom they enjoy conversing. We must do our best to avoid any increase in the patient's feelings of worthlessness when there is evidence that clinical training would be useless because of memory disabilities or senility. Even among this particular group, no one clinical procedure is applicable for every individual other than that of careful evaluative listening.

A reminder—and this is *always* to be kept in mind: many elderly patients have strong positive drives and the neurological ability to regain varied levels of former activities. Hear them out and provide appropriate guidance before you reject them as patients. Any procedure that follows must be based on the specific facts that pertain to each household. Such people are intensely interested in how they may help but can only provide appropriate assistance in the light of objective fact.

Preretirement Years

Those who were employed at the time of their accident are most likely to have a strong motivation toward recovery. The same is true of the stricken housewife because her role is equally important. A significant percentage of these people have not experienced any obvious neurological degeneration prior to their assault. They have, for the most part, a strong desire to reassume their gainful activities. Emotional distractions, however, are extremely detrimental to even the slightest recovery. Again, we must remember that other members of the household can be equally distressed, and if their ambitious drives are unrealistically high, there is a further reduction of possible recovery.

Many find it terribly difficult to reduce their anxious pace without a knowledge of existing facts. There is a subtle conditioning process that influences modern-day expectation. The horse-and-buggy days are gone! The speed of air transportation in itself has reduced tolerance of slower travel; less time is required for general household maintenance; and educational procedures are faster and more intensive. Recovery from many illnesses is now relatively short as a result of new drugs and new procedures. There are few reminders that the basic healing processes are time-consuming, and it is difficult for some families to make realistic adjustments. Time pressure never helped a dysphasic.

We must remind them that it still takes approximately nine months for the female to prepare her infant for delivery and that it will take several years thereafter for the youngster's nervous system to complete its development. Despite our modern drugs and prosthetic devices, broken bones still require prolonged periods of time for mending. These families must be helped to understand that there is rarely a complete recovery from brain damage, and even slight neurological improvements are indeed time-consuming. To date, there is no way to hasten this organic process because unfortunately brain damage is still poorly understood. Neurological pathways in the body below the brain seem to regenerate, but they cannot be rushed nor can the extent of recovery be accurately predicted. This alone should motivate caution on our part and stimulate us to provide repeated consultations for the members of our patients' families.

Spasmodic and brief contacts with the family are of little if any benefit and too often only increase anxiety.

Once you have arranged appointments for family guidance, casually converse with them but avoid dominating the conversation. When we do all the talking and load our expressions with professional terms, additional fears of the unknown are created that merely increase the hopelessness of the family group. Consider yourself for just a moment and estimate the demoralization that you would experience if, as a sophomore, you were enrolled in an advanced postgraduate course but had no language background for the subject at hand. How long could you tolerate such frustration without becoming totally discouraged, irritated, or passive? This trauma can be quickly generalized into over-all behavior patterns. It is contagious and could even interrupt the stability of your roommate or family. Fortunately *you* can escape by dropping the course and enrolling in one better designed for your abilities. We must remember that familial anxieties are even more detrimental since family members have no escape and may actually experience more demoralization than their patient, who has some protection due to the reductions in intellect, memory span, and limited ability to predict the future.

The following may sharpen your alertness to familial problems as they pertain to the patient's welfare. One of our stricken patients, the man of the house, had been totally responsible for the management of all financial affairs. Consequently his wife had little knowledge of the many necessary expenditures nor any experience in budgeting. With no guidance in such matters, this new responsibility itself can create a strong subconscious resentment and eventually disrupt the former positive attitudes toward her husband. We must never blindly *assume* that all is well with the families of dysphasic patients. If the wife makes no reference to financial obligations during her initial visits with you, ask her how things are going. Give her a chance to expose her need for help. You may then suggest or make arrangements for her to contact a family guidance counselor, her banker, a business department in a local university, or even the financial manager of your clinical center. She may appreciate your calling such a consultant for an appointment. Monetary matters are a very personal affair, and very few are willing to reveal details to friends and neighbors. Why should we clinicians involve ourselves in such matters? We can only answer that it may be for no other reason than to show our concern, which if done appropriately will increase the wife's confidence in our sincerity and competence. Most importantly, the solution of such anxieties or hostilities may aid the patient's drive for recovery. We must be cautious however and not rush her and be sure she is willing to expose her financial anxiety before you help to get the assistance she needs.

Eventually most wives will find it necessary to seek employment. Some will have savings, stocks, or insurance, which will reduce the need for full-time employment so that they can continue to visit the clinic. Those who work full time are often given time off for the necessary clinical contacts. This is particularly true if the employer understands the necessity when they are hired. There are but very few instances in which the wives are unable to keep at least one daytime appointment per week. When this is not possible we are professionally and personally obligated to provide evening or weekend appointments. This is not the best arrangement, but it can be done. If a person is willing to keep an evening appointment after working all day, will tolerate the additional expense of hiring an evening attendant for her husband, and will further postpone various home chores, surely we speech clinicians can arrange time for consultations. We have many opportunities to alter our schedule—these wives have none.

As you have probably deduced, the wife of a dysphasic patient does not have an easy role. All sorts of anxieties arise, and we must do our utmost to assist in lessening her tensions and avoid creating added negativisms in her husband's self-attitude. Should she have symptoms of health disturbances, such as weight loss, chronic fatigue, or persistent repetitions of respiratory infections, we should encourage her to acquire medical assistance. Don't offend her—be casual in your suggestion. It would do no harm to contact her husband's physician and report your observations. He may have had but little contact with her because the majority of his time has necessarily been devoted to her husband during scheduled visitations. Remember, the physician is interested, and he will appreciate your attentiveness. He too knows that the state of the patient's mental health depends on those within the immediate environment. Above all, the effectiveness of our clinical procedures depends on her ability to make necessary adjustments. When she is physically despondent we can hardly expect her to be emotionally or intellectually alert. Such behavior is contagious, and her husband already has more than he can handle in isolation.

The discussion thus far is not meant to imply that the *husbands* of stricken wives are comparatively free from anxieties and sincere concern. In fact, they are quite often more traumatized with feelings of guilt because they feel that they must unavoidably neglect their spouses. They have to keep working if only to pay past bills. Very few can consider taking time off for consultations, and when they are at home, most of them are completely lost. Not many have ever made their beds before, let alone done any washing, ironing, or cooking aside from charcoal broiling some meat in the back yard on Sunday afternoons. They may have been almost solely concerned with their jobs. After the wife has suffered the trauma, self-pity may dominate the husband's concerns. He is lost and alone and helpless. Just a little attention from us at such a time often reaps mammoth rewards. Family guidance centers are not extinct, so find one and make a referral. We must help him arrange time to understand his wife's situation more fully. We must make every attempt to contact the people who care for his wife during the day while he is working in order that they too may better understand how to assist her language recovery.

Ideally, the clinical environment should have an apartment-like facility consisting of a small but fully furnished living room, kitchen, and bedroom. The old adage, "Seeing is believing" is accurate if we add "in the light of careful guidance." In unusual circumstances closed-circuit television can provide auditory and visual demonstrations of techniques for language stimulation. This gives the family an opportunity to observe the patient and the language clinician in action. Regardless of the patient's familial role, each of the rooms is adaptable to demonstrations of careful, nondirective language stimulation. The clinician may also observe the patient's reactions to the activities employed by the family members. Helpful guidance is more readily forthcoming when visual observations are provided without distracting the patient's momentary concentration. Such instruction not only benefits the patient; it also enlightens familial insight and security. In addition to independent consultations in the clinic, they may, when it is deemed necessary, bring the patient with them for re-evaluations and specific familial guidance.

Professional personnel in related services may also use the facility to clarify assignments for guidance in the home. When each of us in medicine, speech pathology, psychology, audiology, physical therapy, occupational therapy, nursing, and social welfare has an opportunity to observe these activities as a group, interprofessional staffings are obviously more beneficial. This type of facility is applicable to numerous speech, language, and hearing disorders.[1]

[1] Such facilities are available at the Portland Center for Hearing and Speech, Department of Otolaryngology, University of Oregon Medical School, Portland, Oregon.

EMOTIONAL ATTACHMENTS OF HUSBAND-WIFE

We are readily prone to *assume* that most of our clients have had a satisfactory marital relationship and that it will be retained after the neurological accident. Be cautious, however, in making these assumptions. As we concentrate on any type of speech disorder, it is evident that interpersonal adjustments have an obvious bearing on the success of our clinical procedures. This is particularly true of the dysphasic adult because his progress is relatively dependent on both the pre- and post-traumatic familial relationships. Clinical personnel should have taken an introductory course in marriage and family management. A basic knowledge of this process will assist the detection of subtle disruptions and stimulate referral to a qualified counselor. Each of us has the ability to camouflage our severe dislike of certain people with whom we must associate. We all seem to be born actors, and so it is with some of the familial groups with whom we must work. When marital rejection persists without detection, the patient may have little desire for even the slightest recovery. Conversely, when a patient is overly determined to recover, his major drive may be that of "showing the old lady." It is obvious that this emotional tension can reduce even slight adjustments. Very few people, damaged or not, are capable of satisfactory progress when blind emotionality dominates their every move.

The following case summary will reveal the importance of careful contact with the patient's family *before* he is enrolled for direct retraining. Many tensions can be avoided when such measures are employed.

Mr. X was the chief executive of a large corporation prior to his cerebral assault when he was in his early fifties. His customers and the majority of his fellow workers seemed to have had a profound respect for his executive abilities. Both he and his wife had, at one time, been socially active in their country club, church, and neighborhood. Most of their acquaintances, however, were unaware of his addiction to alcohol. Approximately three years before his illness, a few of his closest business associates observed his alcoholic problem but carefully avoided discussing it even among themselves. A progressive increase of malcontent developed between him and his wife due to the drinking. Their two daughters were in college, and Mrs. X was determined to retain her marital status until the offspring completed their scholastic training. Though Mr. X managed to control his alcoholic illness relatively well during office hours, he made up for lost time at home each evening. As you may suspect, there was a gradual decrease in social contacts outside the home, and his wife became more and more reluctant to voluntarily participate in any joint activities with her husband. Despite this downward pathway there was no indication of marital conflict at home, let alone in public. Unfortunately, the youngsters developed a strong rejection of their father, and it had a negative effect on their own introspection and socialization. Eventually they refused to go home even over the Christmas holidays. This, of course, increased their mother's depression and her antagonism toward her husband. His expenditures on alcohol began to decrease the bank account, which further reduced the familial security. Despite all this deterioration, Mrs. X retained an appearance of sincere and affectionate devotion to her husband. She had no *obvious* symptoms of malcontent.

Suddenly, while at work, Mr. X lost consciousness. Noticing an alcoholic odor, his colleagues quietly took him home and put him to bed. His wife called the family physician when her husband failed to respond to anything some four hours later. He was rushed to the hospital, and it was determined that he was suffering from a cerebral embolism.

You may readily understand the conflicting emotional reactions that persisted among the members of his immediate family, particularly his wife. She had a sincere and capacious concern about his health and a strong desire for his recovery. However, there was continuous anxiety and negativism toward his alcoholism. Mrs. X retained a persistent feeling of isolation from her former friends even though they provided unwavering assistance and devotion.

An excellent health summary was forwarded to a speech clinic, which indicated a progressive neurological recovery but no progress in communication. Medical personnel strongly urged Mrs. X to contact the director of that clinic immediately, but fifteen months passed before she complied. She seemed to have a strong devotion to her husband, and professional personnel were encouraged to believe that he might possibly regain sufficient language for basic needs. Mrs. X agreed to participate in weekly consultations but after her third appointment failed to return, except for transporting her husband to and from the clinic. For the most part Mr. X was excessively congenial, but each time his wife was mentioned, his facial countenance immediately shifted to an obvious expression of "distaste." Despite his clinic visits, he failed to reveal any recovery of language. It became evident that there was no need for the speech clinician to continue seeing him under these circumstances, but that his wife should be referred for psychological or psychiatric assistance. After due consideration the family physician felt that she should be seen by a psychiatrist.

Several months later the psychiatrist forwarded a final clinical summary. The wife had been extremely close to a truly psychiatric depression, which readily accounted for much of her behavior. After she resumed contact with the speech clinician, she voluntarily discussed former anxieties and gradually revealed her husband's history. Even though he was not scheduled for regular appointments, it became apparent that Mr. *X's* communication began to improve immediately. Eventually, he was formally enrolled in the clinic, but the vast majority of professional activities were more supportive than directive. In essence, he was simply given freedom to discuss his interpersonal relationships, and there were no isolated drills on individual words, unless he so requested. Two years later, he had sufficient control to obtain employment through the Office of Vocational Rehabilitation. The vast majority of his intellectual and communication improvements seemed to come naturally once the emotional climate was improved at home. Most families do not have such entanglements, but it is important that we be cautiously thorough in obtaining information before we initiate any therapeutic clinical contact with the patients.

Family members are bound to increase their protectiveness after a cerebral insult, but we must be alert to the possibility that overprotectiveness can also be associated with feelings of guilt. The wife or husband may feel compelled to restrict every activity of the patient, to insist on continuous rest in bed, or even to eliminate any social visits in an effort to lessen feelings of guilt concerning earlier familial conflicts. At the same time, there may also be a feeling that guilt or hostility remains hidden in excessive concern for the spouse's survival and comfort. Regardless of the motivation we are again obliged to contact the physician to determine if there is a need for such stringent restriction of all activities. If not, get the doctor's cooperation in helping the spouse to feel that he or she is now ready to provide more activities that may help the patient's recovery.

Sometimes it helps if we casually discuss the way we ourselves react when we are tired, sick, or emotionally distraught. The following clinical conversation may demonstrate such a procedure: "When we don't feel good it is easier just to sit down and let others assume our obligations. If we are lucky, we won't even have to talk to anyone.

In order to save face, we may very quietly and casually offer some mild objections when others take over our chores, but they will keep going if we really look sick and sound that way. If we have to let them continue over a lengthy period of time, we are relieved of activities that we particularly dislike such as sweeping the sidewalk, pulling the weeds out of the flower garden, or even making up the beds. In essence, none of us really enjoys everything that we have to do, and if there is any possibility of evading certain chores we'll surely take advantage of sloughing-off.

"Of course, we always take a chance when we behave this way. Our family may begin to see that they really don't need us as much as they thought they did. Once we make an effort to resume our activities they may refuse to relinquish some of the most pleasant ones. It doesn't take long for us to show displeasure, and sometimes we say things that really aren't very acceptable. When this happens we get our own way—and more too—they may readily comply and just stop doing anything. Worse yet, we may become isolated because they see no reason to take a chance on any further tirades. This is a very lonesome feeling. We don't enjoy being ignored by those we love the most, but *we* can verbalize our amends. Very shortly, our negative spurt is understood and completely forgotten. Our family resumes their normal behavior, and this enhances our attempts to retain positiveness.

"Now, when we consider your husband it seems possible that he too may react in a similar manner. In other words, he still retains some normal attitudes and will want to do many of the things he enjoyed the most. At the same time he will probably try to avoid participating in activities that he always disliked. It may be a good idea to keep a list of the things he wants to do and then find out if he should go on doing them. If you have any question about his being physically able, you or I can call your doctor for advice. We should be careful and not call him too often though. Perhaps it is better to wait until we have a short list of activities and questions before we contact the physician. In the meantime you can tell your husband what you are doing, and he will probably understand, momentarily at least. When he again insists, just calmly repeat what you told him earlier. He will probably remember that this happened and not be exasperatingly insistent. He too knows that he should be careful, but sometimes he has a hard time remembering his disability."

We must remember though, that the wife tends to be intently aware and fearful of his condition, and we may often have to referee the extreme reactions of husband and wife. There is no need to be dictatorial—there is a need for verbalized understanding.

EDUCATIONAL BACKGROUNDS

Regardless of the educational achievements observed among these families, simple clarity of expression is the tool of utmost importance for the clinician. The basic impression to give is one of cordial acceptance. They already know you are a college graduate, and just this fact may establish a barrier that must be weakened or, better yet, removed. True, we are conditioned to impress our colleagues with our abstract language capabilities, but unfortunately even they have a hard time following us and vice versa. When you go to your physician, dentist, or lawyer do you need help or do you need to be impressed by their abstract prowess? The answer seems obvious; remember it and apply it to your own clinical consultations.

Familial groups are distraught, and this in itself upsets their ability to handle abstractions. I learned my own lesson early and shall always appreciate the honest and frank reaction I received. A physician brought his young child to the clinic where I was pursuing my graduate training. Being terribly impressed with my recently acquired knowledge, I rambled on in the professional lingo of our clinical field. After about five minutes of ego expansion, I was abruptly returned to a state of reality with this remark from the father: "Knock it off! I know you're qualified or I wouldn't have come in. Talk to me as if I were a plain uninformed father so I can benefit from this consultation." Enough said. If this physician had trouble understanding, imagine the importance of simple clarity for the average families of stricken patients. We must speak simply and directly.

Just one more example before moving on. Following my cerebral assault, colleagues here and there assumed that both my wife and I were capable of understanding the abstract language of my profession. My poor wife had learned some of our expressions through her quiet politeness to me and my colleagues, but not enough to follow clearly their abstract ramblings after my accident. I had trouble too. There was some recall of the language they were using but I was acutely deficient in defining their rapidly abstract language expressions. What a relief when they departed! Fortunately some of them could talk simply and plainly; otherwise we would have been completely isolated. Remember, it is necessary that we clinicians be considerate and nourish our lingual egos elsewhere. Concentrate on the purpose of your familial contact and use language that they can understand.

SOCIAL ACTIVITIES

All of us are different and so are the patients who come to us for help. Many of them seem to have energetic moments, but they also have long periods of organic lassitude, and neither extreme is predictable. We must always emphasize this fact when we counsel the family. At the same time we must continually encourage them to provide a variety of opportunities for the patient to get together with friends and neighbors. This indeed sounds contradictory, and it is if we are not careful to stress the necessary flexibility. Close friends are tolerant because they have more affection and ties, but the relationship can dwindle if they are not able to understand broken commitments. We must help the family to explain these disruptions clearly to their acquaintances. The possible demoralization of the patient must always be kept in mind. Fatigue is a major source of depression, and inappropriate or excessive pressure can only add further defects in language acquisition. When a scheduled visit must be cancelled, the patient may wish instead to take a short ride in the car or simply to get out of the house and sit in the yard. If nothing else, this will give him an opportunity to lessen his feeling of guilt or inadequacy and may even erase his internal but false sense of rejection. This is particularly true when others in his household reveal no evidence of disappointment. They won't when they understand that the patient's lack of enthusiasm is not petty protest but based on an organic need for freedom from stress. Sometimes, if it is medically feasible for the patient to be alone, he may feel less guilty if his wife goes on to see their friends while he retires for a rest. It will help her if she can get away for a short time. She, too, will have a rest when she is released from confinement.

It is strongly advisable to postpone dinner parties, even at home, until these patients reacquire sufficient control of the paralyzed musculature or learn to use the nondominant side of the body. But again we must be flexible in our recommendations. It takes a long time for some of the dysphasics to attempt a change in handedness willingly. Our self-concepts often involve the body image.

Family conflicts also often hover in the shadows of social isolation, so it is unwise to expose them too soon. Perhaps, until the patient is able to satisfactorily feed himself, he may be willing to eat before dinner guests arrive. Later, he can join them at the table, have some coffee while others eat, and actively participate in their visit. There are many menus that require little if any need for a knife, thus permitting the patient to join the meal without the tensions of having to fumble with the meat. Mealtime chatter is usually more casual, and there tends to be a better opportunity for the patient to express himself.

Most patients will eventually be willing to exchange visits with close friends after they have once experienced success at home. When this occurs, they have more to talk about. Visits can be overdone though. Brief visits help to overcome detrimental tiredness and consequent negativism. When the patient is ready to leave he will let it be known either verbally or through symptoms of decreased social contact and over-all tiredness. His family should then depart quickly to preserve his willingness for future visits. Even very slight postponements in departure can increase resistance to later contacts away from home. Gradually, the sick one will be physically able to increase the length of social time, but willingness depends on positive experience.

When there are bad times, family anxieties can overflow on the patient if our clinic door is closed or unavailable. Tensions are highly contagious, and they build up when social failures occur repeatedly. If this happens, have the family postpone outside visits until you can hear them out. It will do no harm to suggest that the patient be seen by the physician when he continues to resist visiting; he may be in real need of medical attention.

OFFSPRING IN THE HOUSE

It stands to reason that the children also experience a devastation in their personal security when a parent suffers a cerebral insult. When we fail to take this into account, our professional, let alone personal, efficiency is seriously impaired. Regardless of the children's ages, a sudden organic change in either parent is indeed traumatizing. Children feel these changes keenly. None of us enjoys talking to nonresponsive acquaintances or to those who are hyperirritable or strange and unpredictable. We avoid such persons if at all possible, but once we acquire insight into the reasons for their behavior we often find them tolerable. And so it is with the youngsters of the patient's family. We are obligated to help the nondamaged parent understand the plight of the offspring and thus retain reasonable security for them within the household. Often it is important to counsel the children too.

Young Adults

What about the sons and daughters in their late teens and early twenties? They are just beginning to complete their social and personal independence. Certainly each of us can remember the varied degrees of strife in our late teens. With our first job, we were old enough to pay income taxes but not old enough to vote. We could purchase a car for cash but legally could not acquire credit for the purchase of tires. We were told we had grown up but were immediately pressured to ask permission to go out for the evening. There was love and not-love for those in the household because they had confidence and no-confidence in our abilities. Worst of all, we wanted to leave and yet we didn't because there was still a need for support and control. We were the victims of our own inconsistencies. These are strenuous years for everyone concerned.

These young adults will be as grieved and distraught as their non-damaged parent. A sense of loyalty to both parents dominates their emotions, but as time passes, self-concerns may eventually come to the fore. They may subconsciously focus their own troubled concerns on the patient, who has unavoidably created an alteration in their highway to the stable peaks of independence. Their occasional rejections can be detected by their sick parent, and when this occurs the patient feels further isolation. Even though there may be no intentional condemnations, their discussions often center on the trials and tribulations caused by the illness of their parent. When the dysphasic is unable to participate in these conversations he is the silent recipient of additional hopelessness. Even those dysphasics who are able to express themselves with telegraphic language are too often ignored as they interject apologies and suggest solutions in such situations. So, why should they *try* to regain any verbal usage if they are to be ignored?

We must always do our best to prevent negative discussions among the family group in the presence of the patient. Invite these older offspring to your center, hear them out, and if necessary make appropriate referrals for further assistance. Those who are pursuing an advanced education may obtain financial help from varied governmental or private agencies in their local communities, so refer them quickly. Discuss the stricken parent's condition and help lessen their ignorance and rejection. They deserve the same thorough and cautious attention that is provided for their undamaged parent. Remember, however, most of them have two living parents, and much of their concern may involve both of them. Give them a chance to clear the air before you start total family consultations. Incidentally, the well parent *may also appreciate* an opportunity to vent woes about the children's attitudes. The dysphasic parent will benefit from the self-insights of others at home. As the total family finds solutions to many of their own disruptions and can recognize the do's and don'ts of their contacts with the patient, there will be far more reward for language attempts and an increased sense of being needed.

The Unfortunate Adolescent

Our society seems to have a chronically negative attitude toward adolescents. Perhaps this devastating reaction has always existed. If so, our forebearers must have been more relaxed or at least more accepting of the rugged pathway to stabilized adulthood. Regardless of the social attitudes surrounding them, adolescents are sensitive beings and must not be overlooked. They are a major portion of the constellation, and they have serious concerns for the welfare of each family member. More often than not, the adolescent has a real desire to do the things that their parents expect of them. They want to help and will help if they are regarded as normally stable persons. True, their backlog of experience is limited, but they simply need an appropriate understanding of the problem of dysphasia. They can also assist us to understand the problems of both their parents. Often they provide for the therapist an insightful pathway to follow as he approaches the stricken parent.

We seem to fear the things of which we know the least. Fear can create chronic anxiety, and the latter can stabilize subconscious but habitual neglect. When our patients experience a mysterious avoidance by those whom they love the most, their internal desire for effective recovery can be permanently weakened. The same is true of the offspring if they are not included in our clinical consultations. We must always give the youngsters an opportunity to see us privately to talk about their school work, dances, games, home chores, and general patterns of coexistence with the dysphasic parent. It is amazing how well they can express themselves once they feel secure and realize that we listen with utmost interest. We must not rush it, but at the appropriate time we must raise some questions about the patient's former relationship to them. They will probably be more honest than you suspect possible and will often reveal pertinent interrelationships of their parents. The vast majority of husband-wife interaction is usually positive but may not be mentioned by their mother or father because it has been so habitual and unconscious.

But most of all, the children will want some specific guidance rather than theoretical discussions. They *want* to help.

One of the many parent-offspring tensions is that of deciding on the TV program of the hour. The children usually win out, but their attitudes can be altered once they understand that the stricken parent's favorite program can provide enjoyable language stimulation. Children can learn to accept the post-stroke rigidities. Indeed they often come to enjoy their parent's choice after they are given specific instruction about how to use the varied programs as topics of conversation. We should ask them to help us determine which of the programs our patient enjoyed the most, and then we can use them clinically too.

We must caution them to avoid extensive talk about former physical recreation in which they participated with their stricken parent. Fishing, ball games, camping, hiking, horseback riding, and similar activities may no longer be possible. Even slight references to the things "we used to do" readily defeats positive progress if the patient can no longer be active. Instead we should help the children to determine what kinds of things they now can do with their sick one and help them devise others. We must make them our clinical assistants.

They should also come to understand the importance of regulating the visits of their friends in compliance with the rest patterns of the patient. The patient's welfare must come first. Don't presume that they already understand the why's and wherefore's. We must remember that they may only half hear most of what their parents say. The mother "bosses" but we inform; they are more apt to listen to us and less likely to resent our direction. Our own youngsters resist parental "bossiness" far more than the suggestions of classroom teachers and even neighbors. They know parents too well and really suspect their competence.

In all this counseling we should always explore the many irritations that plague our stricken patients. With our help the youngsters can verbalize and ventilate the many exasperating conflicts in their home. We must help them understand that they are not always at fault, that much of the patient's reactions are uncontrollable, self-condemnatory, and terribly exaggerated. We should ask them to keep a list of such incidents and to discuss them with us. In due time they may better tolerate the patient's involuntary explosions of emotion. We must be both objective and permissive, letting them know that we expect no perfection. As they learn how to control their own outbursts, the patient will be more likely to re-establish improved emotional controls.

The adolescent's observations of anxieties in both parents are usually quite factual, and they provide us with additional topics of discussion with the well parent. Separate counseling sessions can establish appropriate readiness for later total group consultations and most importantly, the air is cleared for positive family-patient interaction in the home environment. The age-old question always persists, "What about those who will not come in or follow through?" The answer is: "Let us do our utmost."

Preadolescents

Extensive changes in familial relationships can drastically affect the youngest children in a family. A well-qualified speech clinician in dysphasia should have a strong minor in clinical psychology to recognize pertinent symptoms of behavioral disruption and refer such children for competent assistance whenever necessary.

Regardless of how hard one may try, there is little that can be done to control rigidly the gyrating activities of *preschool* youngsters. Pressures are not calming nor are they necessary. Young children's attention spans are short, outbursts are brief, and gleeful activity dominates the over-all behavior. A *long* life is in their future. We must do what we can to create optimal conditions for the recovery of our patient, but we cannot remove all stress nor should we create expanded disharmony.

Most of the sick ones value their youngster's affection and attention. They like to hear them talk; they enjoy their children's spontaneous enthusiasm. If nothing else, the verbal expressions are not only enjoyable but stimulating to recovery. The childish chatter does not seem to produce undue strain. Children help dysphasics when they tell them about their activities. Sincere displays of affection from the child provide the patient with a strong sense of being wanted and appreciated. Hardly anything is more positive for the stricken parent's morale than the joyous giggles of the children as they respond to his funny faces or amusing expressions. The patient's language usage is often increased markedly during these pleasurable interactions. Even gesturing helps comprehension and conveys the nuances of effective expression; but most of all, spontaneity thrives on relaxing pleasure in communication.

Another source of pleasure occurs when the child and his parent exchange comments as they turn the pages of an illustrated story book. A word of caution, however—brightly colored pictures are often exceedingly disturbing to the impaired parent. Many preschool booklets have a predominance of pastel colorings, which lessens this stress. Black and white illustrations are even more suitable. It is good for parent and child to observe these together—especially if it provides relief from self-pressures to talk extensively.

Despite favorable and responsive contacts with the young ones, unpredictable spells of fatigue will continue. At times the patient's mate must temporarily distract the young child's attention and get him to do other things so the patient can rest. Yet she must never make the child feel he should avoid contact with the stricken parent. When chronic avoidance develops, the patient loses parental status, language stimulation, and most importantly, the affectionate relationships that are so healing. Most preschoolers take an afternoon "nap." They may not go to sleep; but at least they are confined to their rooms, and the environmental chaos is lessened. This provides relief for the patient to retire quietly or to have an opportunity for isolated chatter with his wife. Most often the conversation in this situation can be initially stimulated with a discussion of the child's activities. When the patient has an opportunity to release regrets, concerning temporary rejections of the youngsters, relationships are often improved after the nap. Remember, simmering negativisms thicken the crust of guilt and can ruin the flavor of objectivity for each and all.

For the most part, children in the elementary school age group can eventually recognize the symptoms of their stricken parent's fatigue, despondency, and subtle irritations. But they need constant help to both acquire and maintain insightful reaction patterns and thus surpass the blunderous chasms of habitual isolation.

ORDERLINESS AT HOME

We must approach the discussion of home orderliness cautiously, particularly when very young children are in the family. It is never easy to tolerate accusations or implications of personal laxity. Sometimes it is helpful for the clinician to apologize casually for the disorder on his desk (if you are abnormal—disorder it before they come in) and to make some remarks about how even this minor confusion often interferes with the attention of the dysphasic clients. This might be followed by remarking that the disorder of your own apartment or home would surely upset your patients. About this time the spouse you are counseling may complain about the litter the children leave throughout the house. If this occurs, you then have an opening, particularly if she implies an appreciation for suggested methods to control their carelessness.

Parental bedrooms are usually off-limits to youngsters, but they do occasionally flutter in. This room, however, will be the major center for the disabled parent throughout long periods of time each day and may continue to be so indefinitely. We must offer suggestions for curtailing the activities of the children within this portion of the home. The stricken ones will also spend considerable time in the living room. Most youngsters can be and are encouraged to use their own rooms for play activities, but again they will stray from these confines. Hence, the living room can become disorderly, but not terribly so; it takes but a moment to clear it up.

The major point of this discussion is to remind us again to *keep reminding* our families of their patient's inability to tolerate disorder easily. Too much stimulation, too much disorder can inhibit positive progress; worse, it can defeat recovery despite prolonged training.

Perceptual problems in the home milieu

The disordered adult does not receive or evaluate the messages of sensation in a normal way. Responses to any stimuli, physical, emotional, or intellectual, are exaggeratedly different from those in the pretraumatic existence. Let us discuss this problem realistically.

Most activities of varied situations perceived by the normal population arise from visual, auditory, tactual, and kinesthetic cues. Normal people are able to sort out substance from shadow and figure from ground. But the brain-damaged cannot consistently perceive the whole of anything. They do not receive the same images of which they were formally aware. Patterning is most difficult. Things are comprehended distortedly. Most patients recognize this but cannot understand their misconstructions of reality. Worst of all, neither do the families or even some of their clinicians. Misconstruction of reality is a basic problem of the dysphasic.

Previous to the accident, the patients could perceive both the whole and its varied details, then choose their pathway of reaction. With brain damage, this ability is suddenly thwarted. They see the whole, but it is fogged with numerous details. Often only one aspect is comprehended, thus resulting in an endless sequence of misconceptions. The following may exemplify the perception of brain damage:

Before his illness, one of our patients was quite sophisticated about automobiles. He readily distinguished between makes, models, and types. This involved both the total forms of the vehicles and minute details of design. After his stroke, there was an inability to clearly perceive anything but the grills on the numerous cars. This particular characteristic is not sufficient for differentiation, but to the patient all cars with "V" shaped grills were made by the same manufacturer. No one could talk him out of it at the moment, and truly, no one should have tried.

After the family understood that he was really seeking a means of getting reacquainted with a disordered world it was easier for them to decrease their insistence of "wrongness." Later, as they took him for automobile rides, the well persons spoke first when they saw autos with the "V" shaped grills. "Oh, there is an Oldsmobile, isn't it, John?" Or, "If I'm not mistaken, that is a Ford." They also then discussed another detail of the car, and their patient most often agreed. Gradually, he became more astute with his perceptions, but it is doubtful that he could have benefited had he been subjected solely to constant correction of his errors.

The perception of totality and the ability to pattern stimulation meaningfully requires continuous but nonthreatening stimulation—not drill books. Formal professional teaching of the "abstract" must always be based on this principle. Human activity is structured by repeated stimulation in the realm of reality. The reorganization process seems terribly gradual, but spurts of progress often occur when a restoration of self-confidence begins to appear.

CONCEPTUAL DISTURBANCES

Most if not all of our dysphasic patients initially lose the ability to generalize. Despite an apparent ability to recall events of interest most accurately, they seem unable to identify them with those similar activities that are removed from specific and current experiences. A very basic example may clarify this disruption. Let us consider the concept "water" in terms of its sources. Rivers, streams, ponds, lakes, the bath, and faucets are a few of our common sources of water. The patient, however, has lost or mislaid the nominal concept of the various origins of water. There is little chance that he will re-establish any usage of these numerous labels unless he has a need for them. Help his family to keep this in mind and yet avoid those undue pressures that create unwarranted sensations of uselessness. Of all the labels listed above, probably the only vitally necessary and meaningful one is the concept of *bath*. Where does one take a bath—in the living room, bedroom, or yard? These are not the places that call attention to *bath* and stimulation for this word in these confines can be terribly meaningless to the patient. It is rather obvious that there is a specific time and place to effectively initiate reuse of the word *bath* and that is in the bathroom itself. Comprehension initially demands a meaningful base that is both useful and appropriately available. So it is with the vast majority of other lingual concepts, i.e., kitchen, food, silverware, tools, and eventually finances and correspondence.

Impress the family group with the fact that they must drastically reduce environmental variations if they are to help their patient recover conceptual formulations. Help them to systematize their activities to bring order out of their patient's chaos. As patterned perception is gradually recovered, it contributes to comprehension, but if either process fades, the other does too. When we are guilty of neglecting the patient's family constellation it is we (all professions) who are to blame for any clinical failures. Remember this before you make unwarranted negative assumptions about your patient's lack of neurological recovery. No patient can see the cause-and-effect relationships when those closest to him are equally uninformed. Drill them to your heart's content if you must, but don't anticipate progress when your patient's family is left without understanding.

DIRECTING ORAL LANGUAGE REFORMULATION

Once the family has a definite understanding that the word *language* has a number of implications, it seems to lessen the pressures that they exert on the patient. Very few people, even among the varied professions, are truly aware of what is meant by language. In the broadest sense it is simply a communicative vehicle of thought. The most basic expressions of language are not dependent on vocalization or specific combinations of speech sounds. Primitive tribes and even some of our American Indians communicate predominately via gesture and grunts that are abstract and symbolic. These are language too; they are meaningful within their own cultures. Profoundly deaf persons express language through an intricate manipulation of body movements. Even our own infants communicate their needs with the basic body postures and vocal wailing.

Damaged adults who have deficits in verbalization are not totally deficient in language usage. Very few have a *total* loss of effective communication. As long as they can communicate with gestures and understand some of the verbal-body expressions of others, there is reason to hope for some degree of progress in reacquiring symbolic communication. We must help their families to understand the significance of all varieties of symbolic communication, to look for them, and to reward them. Unfortunately there is no consistent way to predict the eventual level of verbal recovery other than the response to daily stimulations or careful day-by-day observations. If the patient babbles, at least he is trying to communicate and even this is good. As long as he keeps trying, eventual success may be forthcoming, if his cortex and social environment will allow it.

Families should know that echoic responses are often the first sign of progress. These are the essential base for recovery. Objects and persons represented by these primitive verbalisms are not strongly structured at first because perceptions are not highly differentiated. To the family this is infantile behavior and implies mental deficiency. It may be, but who can really tell? For this reason, if for none other, we must be cautious. False hopes are devastating, but no hope totally eradicates any anticipation of gain. Even though the patient is communciating only with himself and not to others, this may be his way of holding current perceptions and attempting to pattern or stabilize them. His distorted self-talk may be his way of fixing percepts from one experience to the next and may eventually re-establish an orderly arrangement of his understanding. But he must have reward for any effort, and often an objective ear is all the help he needs for several months. This is hard for the families and the clinician, but they must understand. Except for the clinician they probably lack any other person who can or will support their hopes or efforts, and the clinician sees them but rarely.

A number of patients have an extensive but meaningless vocabulary for a long time. They are often unable to organize their language, except for rare occasions during the early stages of recovery. This confusion tends to create emotionality, not only within the patient but also among those surrounding him. It is so easy to lose heart or patience or hope. Negative attitudes are highly contagious and devastating to the basic morale of the total household. We must even help the family to revise their conceptions of the patient's *behavioral* age. True, chronologically he may be fifty-seven years old, but initially at least, intellect and emotionality may appear reduced to a ten-year age level or less. Remember that this often vacillates because there are always instances when he makes sense out of expected nonsense. He may, for two of twenty-four hours, respond maturely. At these times a multitude of hopes arise among those around him, but they fade quickly once his symbolic capabilities lessen or disappear. If his loved ones are not given help in understanding such variations, they may consistently ignore these infrequent but crucial occurrences of their patient's recovery. If this happens there is no reward for the patient's accomplishments, and he too may lose sight of the fact that these slight spurts of normality are possible.

Compare this with your travel along a highway that is under construction. Varied circumstances may have inhibited rapid and total completion of the hardtop surface; the unfinished portion is rough and dusty; travel is terribly slow. Suddenly the hardtop reappears. What a relief it is to stomp on the gas pedal. With no warning, the hardtop is again terminated, and the jolt is alarming. No highway signs exist to warn the driver of the interruption or change. A driver in these circumstances may seek a hardtopped side road, and when one appears quickly take advantage. What a shame if it leads nowhere. Had he stayed on the main highway he could have avoided hours of lost time because only one-half mile beyond his turn-off, the highway was completed. So it is often with the family of a dysphasic. If we can warn them and help them over the rough spots, their patient's road to recovery may become smoother with time.

Automatic responses

All of us use pet phrases, slang, or perhaps "cuss-words" during our daily conversations. Most of the time *we* don't hear it and most of our friends ignore it. They listen to *what* we are saying, not to *how* we are saying it. But beware of their reactions when brain damage is involved. For months inappropriate automaticisms and expressions will punctuate one's speech attempts. The unrealistic anxieties among listeners as their ears pick up these expressions will inhibit initial recovery.

So it is with the majority of the stricken persons. Neither they nor their families can control their automatic utterance. No regulation of listener reactions can exist unless they understand that these uncouth or blatant responses are not intentional. The patient's phrases flow without conscious planning and are unheard as the words are uttered. However, when the patient observes the facial expressions of his listeners, it becomes evident that once again he has failed to communicate his thoughts or has said something wrong or shocking. He may immediately try again, this time becoming aware of some of what he says. If he does detect the ugly or inappropriate expression it shocks him terribly, but if his listeners are calm, he may not give up all attempts to relay his thoughts. Each time he tries, it may or may not improve, but at the very least his own curiosity concerning the listener's responses is more likely to be satisfied. Positive self-awareness even of his mistakes is less detrimental to the patient's morale than shocked and mysterious rejection by his listeners. When he hears what he is saying and if those around him are not upset, he will likely continue to try to talk.

The clinician, when this problem occurs, must be careful to provide careful, positive, and factual information to the family. Because the patient is swearing it does not mean that he is angry or terribly upset at the moment. He may merely be trying to talk. He only becomes disturbed when he senses rejection in his listener. Many of these patients have never sworn in the presence of even the immediate family. In some instances, neither the family nor their distant acquaintances have formerly heard the patient's use of foul language. Let us illustrate: A very fine man, who was the pastor of a large congregation for twenty-five years, was suddenly stricken during his Sunday morning sermon. He uttered some rather profane words just prior to losing consciousness. Absolutely no one had ever *heard* him swear before his accident. Imagine his plight in recovery when even his wife strongly rejected him for profaning the Lord's temple. Many months passed before he could begin to control his swearing. Who was in dire need of immediate guidance—the patient or his wife? After many weeks, she began to speculate on how the swearing vocabulary may have been developed. Both she and her husband had continuous contact with missions in the lower areas of a large metropolis. The language of its despondent and alcoholic population was both uninhibited and emphatic. Some cortical absorption of that language was unavoidable, and when the inhibitory areas of her husband's brain were damaged, it is possible that the oral expressions of profanity were then released. She also admitted that she, herself, had sworn quietly for a number of years and feared similar oral expressions should she be damaged. How many of you reading this treatise would be free from such a possibility were you to have a cerebral insult?

There are other verbal automaticisms, of course, besides cursing, that may also dominate expression. Brief but repetitive phrases, meaningless words, or even portions of poetry learned during childhood may appear again and again. One of our patients had spent several years training personnel for a technical career. Much of the language and varied processes were rather vague to the neophytes with whom he had contact. He meaningfully and most appropriately checked on their understandings of his expressions with the query, "Are you with me?" Following an embolism, the question became automatic in all communicative situations. If he desired a cigarette he would say "Are you with me?" The persons around him rejected the phrase and told him so. He gave up all attempts to talk. Even his gestures were terminated, and it took several months to remotivate any attempt at oral communication. Had the persons who rejected his response been forewarned, recovery could have been less traumatic. Remember again, the patient's recovery is highly correlated with familial insights.

LANGUAGE STRUCTURE

The notion of language retraining, stimulation, or attempts to recall does not mean that grammar should be stressed in guiding the dysphasic until late in treatment if ever. It depends on the background and capacities of each individual. Grammar is the organization of linguistic expression. Grammatical confusion is conspicuous among most brain-damaged adults because the essence of the disorder is confusion in symbolic patterning. Grammatical rules are best learned as babies learn them—indirectly. Rules help little because the irregularities of our language pose an additional handicap. Many words sound alike but refer to different things. Even phonetic relationships vary and create further confusion for the patient. It is difficult for any adult to learn a new language; it is terribly hard to do so if the pedagogy is formal.

Sometimes the language deficiency interferes with the patient's accurate assessment of others, attitudes toward himself. When this occurs, and it frequently does, the family needs to restate the subject clearly after a pause or again with a different sequence of words. Most of the time this helps, but they should know that it can also fail, particularly in the shadows of needless pressure. The patients are not totally insensitive to their lack of comprehension even though it may not show. Stimulations are as effective as the tone and intensity of the speaker's voice. Sharp impatience is useless except for relief of the speaker's inner tensions. It only increases the patient's sense of failure.

Gesturing often clarifies the meanings of oral expressions. This is true of both the patient and the person with whom he is communicating. As he gestures, so should his respondent, because it helps enrich an understanding of the abstract. Again, remember that the original process of language comprehension and development, among infants, depends largely on accompanying body movements. Help the family to be as kind to the dysphasic as they have been with any other beginner. Have them observe your professional activities, and then you should observe their applications of your practices. Together the clinician and the family must determine the appropriateness of pathways to effective stimulation. There is no one formula for all constellations of dysphasia. Each patient presents a unique problem. Moreover, no one patient or family remains static. Variations will occur; we must be alert and use them to facilitate recovery.

IN ESSENCE

Depression among brain-damaged patients is neither a fleeting nor even a casual state of emotional deterioration. It is persistently serious, and it takes extensive time to lessen their demoralizations. These people are *organically* confused and distraught. When abstract clinical training for communication is started before despondency is lessened, it is very rarely beneficial; most individuals become more withdrawn and less productive.

None of us has learned to survive or even approach any level of self-confidence in isolation. Even the most brilliant people in our society must rely on the insights of others to accomplish their tasks in an orderly manner. Clinical personnel are highly dependent on total family and interprofessional thoroughness. When we join the patients' race for social survival we must first assist in the remedy of basic familial anxieties and resulting prejudices. These block the highway to positive recovery and no abstract surface of isolated language stimulation can survive interprofessional blindness. Positive stakes are precious—but they can disintegrate if they are soaked with negativisms in idle assumption.

HAVING JOINED OTHER FELLOW PATIENTS ON THE RUGGED PATHWAY from a cortical insult, the senior author finds it necessary to join them in questioning some of our common professional views. Let us first consider the so-called varieties of aphasia. Many classifications of aphasia appear expressly designed to lessen or even terminate whatever chances for behavioral progress may be present. How *should* we classify linguistic losses or reductions? Can we ever really be sure that the reduction of ability in *oral expression* represents a lesser severity of impairment than the *ability to understand* the utterances of others, or the opposite? Can we ever be certain that our friends are really following our conversation until they make an appropriate response? Can any professor really know that his students are getting his message unless they recite in class or pass written examinations?

5 *evaluation, prognosis, and management of language*

Wouldn't it upset you terribly if you were graded solely on the professor's idle speculation that you do or do not know that which you have heard or read? Yet many dysphasic patients are misevaluated in their receptive ability merely because they cannot respond.

10 For a fairly comprehensive historical review of concepts of aphasia, see Schuell (17) and Klingbeil (10).

The patient's survival is precarious enough without the added anxiety caused by unwarranted clinical suppositions. Unless the categories of language reduction are supported by unwavering facts, the diagnosis may lead to clinical behaviors on the part of the therapist which will thoroughly confuse the patient.

COMPLEXITY OF REDUCED EXISTENCE

As we have seen, the complex network of neutral pathways within the hemispheres of the brain prohibits isolated damage to any *one* aspect of behavior. When there is a deficit in language expression, there is also inevitably a modification in the understanding of language uttered by other persons. So it is with personal adjustments and intellectual functioning, as shown in reading and writing and the other symbolic processes. Many specific reductions in comprehension or expression are variable from day to day. On Monday the patient may make sense when he talks to you; on Tuesday he not only fails to speak sensibly but even appears to lack the comprehension he had shown before. He varies more widely than we do, but we vary too in our ability to communicate.

Most stricken patients retain some ability to use language. Those few who show no evidence of spontaneous recovery in language may do so merely because they have failed to regain sufficient energies to do more than exist. The problem presented by these patients is always global, not partial. The interrelationships between reductions in language, emotions, intellect, and health must be continuously in the minds of all professional personnel who work with the dysphasic. Professional persons in all areas of rehabilitation need assistance in detecting potential function that has been hidden or overlooked. And all of them must be very wary of tagging the patient with diagnostic labels that may not be deserved. Otherwise the patient will be again insulted. For this latter reason, if none other, only one major label seems necessary to categorize the trauma: DYSPHASIA—*a combined disturbance in communication, intellect, emotional stability, and overall health.*

How then shall we evaluate the problem presented by a patient with dysphasia? We find it wiser to begin with some simple questions. "Is the reduced comprehension a result of (1) anxiety and depression, (2) intellectual devastation and deficit, (3) predominantly, a result of damage to the cortex leading to reduction in language controls, or (4) a combination of all of these?" At the present time we are unable, usually, to isolate any of these factors with precision. Until we can be sure, beyond any doubt, that the problems in vocabulary reception are solely the result of a specific cortical destruction, it seems most advisable to refrain from any rigid classification. Too often our diagnostic labels blind us to the true state of affairs and prevent further objective investigation. Consequently, by our diagnosis we often defeat the patients' efforts to recover.

It may be true that those who worry not, recover not, and some patients show no self-concern at all. They are the hebephrenic aphasics, always jolly. Either end of the continuum of anxiety is detrimental to recovery. How do normal people try to protect themselves from revealing their felt weaknesses? One technique is that of incessant chatter. By dominating the conversation with this chatter we keep others from recognizing our inadequacies—we hope. Most of us have done just this at certain times. Though our listeners are undoubtedly bored by our gabbing, we often feel safer in the flood of verbal trivia. It is possible that this kind of behavior carries over or even expands after brain damage. Numerous patients have told us that they have often done this. I, too, employed such a defense when shortened attention spans raised their devastating heads. It made me *feel* better to camouflage my sense of futility with chatter. I felt a compulsive need to control my listeners, and even though I knew it was uncomfortable for them, I felt safer in rambling on. My listeners often seemed to feel that I didn't know what I was doing. They felt compelled to interrupt me and wore me out with silly reiterations of what I had said, whether it made sense or not. Or they would ask me a silly question, or change the topic. Each time there reactions occurred it left me with but one choice—complete silence. Despair then reigned and stimulated immediate withdrawal from communicative interaction. When my professional colleagues responded in this way, I had to flee home, where my neighbors and members of my family permitted more freedom for these expressive ramblings. There I was told that most of my apparently random verbosities had strong traces of sense when they really listened.

Far too often, we impede the dysphasic's potential progress with unrealistic pressures and useless drills, administered too soon. We should avoid the enrollment of any patient for routine language training until after his physician finds real evidence of over-all progress in health, until the psychologist has determined improvement in personal and intellectual abilities, and when the family has reported positive progress in social adjustment. Why must we hurry? The dysphasic is very susceptible to time pressure.

Brain-damaged people are bound to exhibit their egocentricity. This is to be expected, and we feel that it is truly justifiable. These patients were self-centered *before* their accident; without some egocentricity none of us could survive the pressures of normal existence. We are merely able to mask our egocentricity better than the dysphasic can. Moreover, a brain-damaged person must give priority to his own needs. He must survive. This is why he is more concerned with concrete situations than abstractions. Motor and sensory deficits jeopardize personal safety, and survival comes first. It supersedes any drive for social recovery. If dysphasic patients are pushed into formal language training before they adjust to their physical deficits, motivation is lost, resistance is found, and every aspect of concern for social recovery will be diminished or, worse, destroyed.

Many patients experience chronic and severe headaches. This is often undetected by the therapist or companion when they are unable to describe their pains. Enrollment in the language clinic will be of no value to a person whose head feels as though it might explode. We should always be alert to this possibility, ready to refer him to his doctor. Headaches can be dangerous symptoms, and immediate medical treatment may prevent the threat of recurrent damage. Even though the patient may try to respond to the elaborate testing procedures regarding oral language, reading, and writing, it is very doubtful that the results obtained will be very meaningful until after he has a reduction in anxiety concerning his basic survival.

Continuous Evaluations

How long should we wait to test the patient's language and intellectual abilities after the cortical episode? It is impossible to establish a specific time for all patients because even those with the least damage show wide variations in automatic recovery time. Furthermore, we are truly unable to define "automatic" or "spontaneous recovery." Some people are bathed in verbal stimulation, others get very little encouragement, and there are those who receive no help at all. Each patient is an entity both unto himself and his home environment. We must remember that the trauma of dysphasia is always entwined with a lasting and profound emotional shock. Negative emotion can interfere with and prevent language recovery and social readjustments despite anatomical recovery. Some patients are said to have a simple impairment. When we carefully consider each patient's altered self-concept, his weakened energies, and familial and social disruptions, it is difficult to ever use the word "simple."

Any evaluation should be postponed until after the patient is comfortably secure in the clinical environment, and we must remember that he cannot be acclimated quickly. He lives as a stranger in a strangely abstract world, and any threat to his minimal security is indeed traumatizing. It usually takes a matter of several weeks for the patient to relate comfortably to any person outside his family. Until this anxiety begins to subside, clinical judgments based on tests or single observations can be terribly misleading. It takes considerable time for the patient to *show* his potentials. It takes a very gifted clinician to examine these patients—one who is experienced, humane, and relaxed.

Be sure that the family knows also that it will take many people and much time to complete the diagnostic procedures. If the family is aware of the need for lessening pressures, its members will become more relaxed and supportive.

Evaluative procedures should always be programmed in compliance with the individual patient's over-all condition. Dysphasic people tire quickly, and if they are pushed beyond their energies they fail miserably. Many will attempt to resist their own fatigue to the edge of total collapse. Their anxieties are often beyond reasonable self-control, and they can't modify their own compulsive drive for rapid recovery. Visits should be limited to a maximum of thirty minutes, and it is also advisable to see these people during the morning hours before fatigue sets in. Consult with the family before you begin each session. If the patient had a restless night or other troubles, responses can become meaningless. If he is emotional, the patient's attention span will be limited and his responses unrepresentative of his potential.

Identical psychological surveys should be repeated every two to three months throughout the first two years following the patient's accident. In this manner we can evaluate progress in (1) memory and recall; (2) vocabulary expansion and retention; (3) problem solving; (4) behavioral adjustments; and most importantly (5) the patient's reactions to regular instruction in language. The survey procedures must always be meaningful to the patient and undue stresses avoided in the diagnostic sessions. The dysphasic has enough stress of his own.

Let us now consider the question of articulation as it relates to diagnosis. Any reduction in receptive functioning of the tongue and the lip areas will interfere with the clarity of speech. Slight degrees of sensory loss are extremely difficult to detect, particularly when the patient is unable to clearly describe his problem, and this deficit seems to increase with extended fatigue. When the patient's tongue and lips begin to feel sluggish, his interest in language usage dwindles, and any amount of clinical stress opens the door to depressive withdrawal. To him, his articulation sounds as bad as his sensory deficit feels. You will never convince him to the contrary. You must believe him and react accordingly. This feeling of sluggishness and imprecision seems to last incessantly. A number of patients, who have been as fortunate as I in over-all recovery, have described similar experiences. At the end of each day my entire right side (tongue, lips, face, arm, and leg) feels as though it has gone to sleep. It takes more time to walk, to talk. My verbal utterances are slower, vocal intensity is subconsciously reduced, and participation in all conversations lessens. Once, unbeknown to me at the time, my evening utterances were recorded. Upon hearing the recordings I recognized that there was actually no reduction in the clarity of my articulation, but despite this fact, I am still convinced each evening that my speech sounds as sluggish as my tongue and lips feel. Does it not seem obvious that those patients who are in the early stages of recovery are bound to become terribly upset when this occurs? Any person who has experienced a sudden incompetence of language and intellect is bound to retain many self-doubts concerning his recovery, and he tends to trust his feelings more than the reassurances of others.

How Normal Is Normal?

There are many cases in which intellectual and linguistic recoveries have surpassed the patient's ability to control his emotional reactions. Such people may not reveal any deficit on simple language tests; intelligence scores may be close to or identical with pretraumatic records; and there is no outstanding reduction in physical movement. Their families are told that all is going well, and they believe it. Everyone believes it except the patients. They know it is not so, but no one hears their concerns. Such patients are perhaps overly aware of even slight repetitive expressions; they recognize the variations in memory span; many of them sense an awkwardness in muscle movements; and they are acutely aware of sensory changes throughout the stricken half of the body. They know, as no one else can, the effects of their sudden attacks of severe fatigue. They know the loss of personal security. They know the anxiety.

Dysphasic patients often reveal an exaggerated sense of anxious guilt. This is largely due to the fact that too many people expect and want them to act normally. The harder these patients try to fulfill these expectations and desires the more they recognize and magnify their failures. Irrelevancies and inadequacies in language increase; hence, relationships with other people are adversely affected. Such a person may also gradually come to misconstrue what has been said to him and so fail to respond appropriately. Erratic language usage can create an endless array of difficulties in communicating with family members, friends, and fellow workers. The dysphasic cannot comprehend or accept the reasons for his minor failures. He has no recourse except demoralization, frustration, rage, or withdrawal from interpersonal contacts.

Oddly enough, the closer the patient is to being normal, the more he needs *supportive* assistance. Such a patient is alert enough to recognize his abstract deficiencies easily. Even very minor deficits are evaluated as extremely severe because he is now oversensitive. It is terrible to be "almost normal" particularly when even those closest to him lack an understanding of his plight. He needs freedom to complain; to hear himself discuss his internal anxieties; and to drain off his exaggerated concerns long enough to clear the air. He needs supportive guidance. The more *you*, as a therapist, will listen, the less his family and fellow workers will need to be subjected to his worries. In due time, he will be more able to tolerate his minor deficits in utterance or comprehension. He will also come to accept that even his normal acquaintances are not consistently competent in listening and speaking. As his perfectionism subsides, his remaining abilities increase. Thus, those with whom the patient associates should do their utmost to accept his occasional language difficulties casually. With good friends, good clinicians, and a good family that understands, the patient is freed from his terrible isolation.

BASIC LANGUAGE EVALUATIONS

It will be helpful to keep our own limitations in mind if we wish to understand the patient's usual negative reactions to his examination and therapy. Often both appear senseless to the dysphasic. Would we find it pleasurably or beneficially stimulating to attend abstract advanced classes in entomology? Most of us are unable to define entomology nor can we understand the vocabulary used by people discussing its esoteric aspects. In essence, in such a class we would feel "dysphasic" because we could neither understand nor discuss these technical matters. If we were forced to attend such classes repeatedly we would find it impossible to avoid spells of frustration, depressive rage, and intellectual withdrawal. The abstract language in research reports of speech pathology is terribly difficult to tolerate even for many clinicians.

EDUCATIONAL AND VOCATIONAL BACKGROUNDS

We must be especially cautious to use a vocabulary that is commensurate with that of each patient's pretraumatic usage. Those individuals who had achieved a university education expect you to recognize it and talk accordingly. Even though much of the vocabulary may *appear* to the clinician to be too abstract for your dysphasic patient, we should never assume that it is until after the patient so indicates. You should not talk baby talk even to a baby. His self-concept is important, and his ego is deflated enough without having to face being talked down to in a patronizing fashion. After there are repeated evidences of a lack in verbal comprehension we then should modify our expressions, but not before we are relatively certain that the patient truly needs such carefulness.

Spoken phrases of course must be short and, if need be, casually repetitive when we observe that the patient finds it difficult to follow the topic under discussion. Before phrases are repeated, however, be careful to allow plenty of time for responding. If he fails, repeat the phrase again and aid it with appropriate gestures, and facial expressions. Interestingly enough, a number of "wordless" clients often come forth with a surprising amount of language once they are convinced that the clinician is patiently polite and willing to wait them out.

Many patients who feel themselves less educated tend to be somewhat distraught when in the company of a clinician. They react much the same as we do when surrounded by business executives, administrators, and outstanding performers in the arts. In such a situation it seems safer for us to listen rather than join in verbal exchanges. We find it hard to respond voluntarily until after we are sure that it is safe to do so. Dysphasic patients are equally cautious. They need assurance from their clinicians of their acceptance before they will respond.

Many of our evaluative successes will depend on relating the topics of the communication to the patient's former interests and vocation. If you should have a client who had been a waitress, it will be wise for you to investigate the general mode of conversation among the employees of such an establishment. Take your coffee breaks while sitting at the lunch counter where the workers seem to congregate, noting the topics of discussion and the mode of verbal expression. Engage the waitresses in conversation, learn to "talk like they do" and you will learn how to talk to your client. Should your waitress patient have been employed locally, go to that restaurant and engage her fellow-workers in a casual conversation. Let them know of your acqaintance with the patient and ask them for help. Find out how they viewed her; what her recreational interests seemed to be; get their impressions of her apparent level of alertness to the job. All this information will be essential in your clinical activities.

Should one of your clients be a former architect, again investigate his specific working interests. Seek assistance from a high school teacher or university professor of architectural drawing; ask for references to the introductory literature that describes the drawing materials necessary for this professional pursuit. Know what the T-squares, triangles, varied compasses, and drawing boards are *before* you initiate evaluative contacts with your patient. Better yet, visit his former place of employment and strike up an acquaintance with his closest associate. Note the way he talks and about what. Ask for some help in determining the kinds of pursuits your patient *enjoyed* the most.

It may even be helpful if the client's fellow-worker joins the patient in a few of the diagnostic sessions. This will not only improve your understanding but will likely stimulate some expressions of language that may never be forthcoming during isolated appointments. Remember this: many of your patients have been as engrossed in their working activities as you and your own colleagues. When we join our colleagues in social activities we often regress to shop talk and professional chatter. Make use of shop talk with your stricken persons. Such stimulus words as *apple, saucer,* or *fork* are of little value in language stimulation, and most of the material used in the formal tests may be viewed by your patient as insulting and demoralizing. Would you graciously accept such verbal stress if you were dysphasic?

Suppose your patient is a housewife. Again you should investigate her former activities and interests. Visit with a member of her bridge club, talk to her close neighbors and most certainly those within her familial group. Invite them to visit your center with their patient. Observe their verbal interactions so you can capitalize on them during later contacts with the patient. Parenthetically, just because these patients are women, it doesn't necessarily mean that *needle, iron,* or *oven* are the words they need. They may have never used or liked any of them.

Regardless of the level of formal schooling, education is a continuous process. Even if your patient dropped out of high school, he may have major intellectual interests. Newspapers, magazines, television, radio, travel, and recreational pursuits contribute to our growth and shape our interests. For this reason, if none other, we must carefully maintain continuous contact with the patient's family and friends. These people are likely to be aware of the patient's past ability to retain information and to know his varied levels of enjoyable interest. You may be surprised.

Recreational Interests

Many people work solely for monetary survival. Their only real interest in the job is pay day. Dysphasic patients who were employed in a laundry, gas station, delivery service, or grocery store may readily resist any talk about their former occupations. They may have hated their jobs. Instead, their main interest in life may have been centered on recreational pursuits. If so, let's talk about them in our casework. Even though an enjoyable hobby, such as fishing, sewing, or woodcraft, may not be immediately possible, past memories or future hopes about them may readily stimulate a flow of language that would otherwise be forever hidden from us. Contact the personnel in physical medicine. If you will share your observations with them and together estimate the possibility of the patient's modified return to these physical pursuits, the patient may show surprising growth in communicative and physical adaptations. If a patient has a real desire to recover so he can find life desirable, he will be more likely to follow interprofessional guidance. We must remember that there are many good one-handed marksmen, piano players, craftsmen, and even seamstresses. These patients' avocations often become their post-traumatic vocations when their clinicians are alert to such a possibility. Most of all, dysphasics find a reason for communication if they become involved in activities that are enjoyable and rewarding.

Automaticisms

A majority of the dysphasic patients demonstrate some automatic verbal expression, and these phrases or single word utterances may be the first to be spoken after the initial trauma. When this occurs, there is an immediate reward. Their listeners are delighted. The response is highly rewarded. Such a reaction may be a partial explanation for the habitualization of the patient's automatic utterances. Initially, it is almost impossible for these patients to factually evaluate the reactions of persons around them. Even though there may be a predominance of negativism, as when profane interjections are used, it often seems to have but little meaning. The patients have elicited attention and may truly have little concern about the actual evaluations of their listeners.

In due time, however, many seem able to detect society's rejection of their automatic utterances but despite such awareness are unable to alter their language. Why? First, they may simply be unaware of what they are saying. Their own words are as meaningless to them as the vocalizations of others. The deciphering mechanism seems to be absent until they are able to interpret the behavior of their listeners and become aware of their own failures. Then, not only do they retain the verbal automatisms that were conditioned by reward, but they also begin to habituate fearful withdrawal from attempts at any vocalization lest the punishable utterances come forth. When this occurs, everyone with whom they have contact may unwittingly increase the patient's social isolation. Even clinical personnel are guilty of such behavior, and consequently the patients are dumped into a complete social vacuum. As a result of social rejection and withdrawal, the patients have little, if any, opportunity to alter the automatic expressions let alone to expand their ability in understanding the words of other persons.

A severely impaired patient had been hospitalized in a locked psychiatric ward for some twenty years. His only utterance was "Goddam Joe," but he had a variety of vocal inflections. It could sound like "Good morning," "I am fine," "Thank you, sir," or "Goddam you!" In due time, I became fairly accurate in my interpretations of his varied vocal inflections. Unless he was truly irritated, he had been unaware of what he was actually verbalizing. He heard it then and consistently blushed and lowered his head. I seriously doubted that he should be considered seriously psychotic as others had diagnosed him. He was always neat in his personal appearance and kept his own bed and belongings in good order. He was, however, a very lonesome man on that psychiatric ward. Other patients were talking nonsense; they seemed to have no concern with their own appearance nor did they relate to their fellow patients. Their auditory and visual hallucinations created almost total isolation from their associates and certainly provided no stimulus for "Joe" to alter his own automatic verbalizations. The ward attendants, nurses, and physicians rarely conversed with him—this type of isolation was to be expected on that particular ward. The man with his dysphasia was hidden behind the label of "organic psychosis."

A psychological re-evaluation was requested and was the first to be administered during a fifteen-year period. Intellectually the patient was within the mid-normal range as determined on performance, not verbal, tests. Behaviorally, he had strong symptoms of depression and overt withdrawal, but he also revealed some realistic self-concerns. In this case, the habitual isolation from fellow-patients was indeed a matter of self-protection and not a psychiatric problem.

An interprofessional staffing was established, and after due consideration, he was transferred to an "open" ward. There he was given an opportunity to visit the hospital stores, mingle with patients who could converse with him, and most of all he could be among members of the staff who were not unrealistically biased by the prior label of severe psychosis. There was an immediate expansion in his oral vocabulary. At the dinner table he began to ask for "goddam meat," goddam bread," and "goddam coffee." He asked for and bought his own "goddam" Luckies, matches, shaving soap and other articles. Within a period of six weeks even his automatic profanities became less obvious and heightened his personal contacts with fellow patients and the professional staff.

Automatic responses are not necessarily confined to swearing. Such statements as "Well see now," "Thank you very much," and "Good—good, hear this," may unconsciously be emitted, fixed through reinforcement, and often retained in combination with conscious utterances. All of us are guilty of certain verbal automatisms, but we seldom recognize them. Should you experience similar brain damage, you too would be likely to retain utterances of certain phrases. You don't hear them now, and it is doubtful that you would following a cortical assault. Furthermore, a self-examination of our own utterances may readily alter negative reactions to our clients once we recognize our own "dysphasic" behavior. We all often forget words, fail to understand, and speak confusedly.

Evaluating Communication Levels

Despite all the research, there is unfortunately no one test, or group of tests, applicable to each and every patient. Remember your own reactions to academic inquisitions, especially to those tests administered without warning. In most instances your dysphasic clients will be even more traumatized by any kind of formal testing procedure. Just the trip to the testing room is threatening enough without the added apprehension concerning test failure. It is always advisable to postpone formal testing until after the patient has made several visits to your office, and comes to know and trust you. After he has become acquainted with the physical environment, has had an opportunity to become acquainted with both the clinician and other persons concerned, the test results may be more meaningful. However, they are continuously questionable.

11 A description of diagnostic therapy as opposed to one shot testing is provided by Van Riper (21).

When these conditions have been satisfied and the patient seems secure and relaxed, it is wise to begin by brief discussions of the activities that may be forthcoming. Ask for any comments or suggestions that the client may have concerning the nature of his difficulty. Let him know that he is a directive part of the remedial procedures; incidentally incorporate simple explanations of the varied aspects of communication difficulty to show that you understand. In this manner the patient will recognize your respect for him as a person with troubles, particularly if he is given an opportunity to vent his woes and to establish a relationship. No one has the right to test him to utter despair.

In evaluating his responses, put your pen and paper aside. The success of your evaluation depends completely on your cordial attention to the patient's attempts at communication. Any of us would be terribly distracted if the person with whom we are conversing would persistently scribble during our utterances. Moreover, a dysphasic patient becomes fearful and afraid to say anything when threatened with a permanent record of his chatter, especially when he cannot remember what he has said. The written recording of test results comprise an overpowering threat to the language-impaired individual.

Modern recording equipment is no longer massively bulky. Transistorized tape recorders fit our desk drawers, and a good microphone can be camouflaged easily, thus avoiding the distracting threat. After each clinical visit there is an immediate opportunity to analyze the patient's language usage more thoroughly. It is always wise to keep some of the tapes in the patient's file for future analysis of possible language improvement. Recovery is a slow process, and progress is often overlooked without comparative recordings. Progress, over a period of time, is often dramatically revealed by these recordings. They can be invaluable later in bolstering the patient's morale when he can hear the changes that have occurred. Let us say again that isolated formal tests often have but little meaning when compared with unstressed communicative behavior. They are convenient for the clinician and often disastrously unfair to the patient.

If you must write, keep your notebook out of the patient's sight and do your utmost to retain eye contact with him while he responds to your questions. Also record descriptions of his other behavior, such as meaningful facial expressions and gestures. Always bear in mind that the slightest distraction can completely erase his trend of thought. *You are not testing his resistance to chaos; you are trying to determine his basic language needs.* When we are careful to consult with the family before we begin to evaluate the patient, our impressions become more meaningful. The most reasonable starting point is to begin by stimulating his responses to inquiries dealing with his biographical background such as: (1) where he lives and a description of the home; (2) who lives there; (3) who his neighbors are and what they do for a living; (4) whether there are young-sters in the home; (5) if the offspring are married, where do they live? (6) what his hobbies are; and (7) what are the dietary likes and dislikes and numerous other topics related to personal activities.

Should the patient be unable to respond meaningfully to the preceding stimuli, try to elicit responses to naming common articles and surroundings, such as clothing, or the clinic furnishings. Determine the kinds of errors. Are the utterances relatively meaningful? Are the responses totally nonsensical? Are they inconsistent in that there are times when the responses to identical questions are accurate and other times when they are unrelated? Give the patient a chance to make voluntary utterances and note the relevancy to the topic at hand. And give him time!

Again, I remind you to be casual, to avoid stress in pressuring for immediate verbalization and most of all, stop all testing activities before fatigue sets in. Remember that the most important aspect of your contact with the patient is to build a comfortable rapport. Unless he is confident that you truly respect him without condemnation there is little chance to get a fair diagnosis, and you may impede communicative recovery.

I strongly question the common belief that *most* of the spontaneous recovery will occur within three months after the initial assault to the brain. The nervous system is just too complex to support such a dogmatic assumption. Who can see into the brain? We cannot set any arbitrary time limit on recovery. There are too many "goddam Joes" who have been professionally ignored because of such unfounded speculation. True, some patients do progress rapidly during the first weeks and then slow down. But there are many others who show no progress for several months, and yet, with time, frequently surpass those who excelled immediately after the trauma.

The clinician's daily logs will often be far more meaningful than any formal tests viewed in isolation. Test results on one day may be markedly different from those obtained on other days, and little can be predicted from them until after relative stabilization occurs. Even stable patients reveal obvious variations in their language performance. On one occasion a patient may refer to his wife *Mary* as *Mary*; name *socks* as *shoes* and the *window* as *door*. The following day he may refer to his wife *Mary* as *the woman* or even by his daughter's name *Carol,* the *shoes* as *shoes,* and the *window* as *sun.* Even during the course of writing this text, six to ten years after my thrombosis, I have known occasional episodes of nominal confusions. Written errors were not detected until I reread the script the following week. This exemplified a dysphasia both expressively and receptively. Had I been tested during these times I would indeed have acquired a label of "moderately severe dysphasia." Yet, on the majority of days, the results would have indicated normality. I am neither totally dysphasic nor am I totally normal. *Broad labels are bound to be inaccurate.*

To avoid the usage of single-word diagnostic labels, it is wiser to describe day-to-day consistencies and inconsistencies. Any behavior, verbal or not, seems to have varying peaks of efficiency. Remember that all reaction is a process operation, not a statistically predictable occurrence. The most minute variations may often become major contributions to the process of recovery. The pattern of progress is, of course, very gradual and more apparent month-to-month than week-to-week, and particularly day-to-day. Any conclusion from a one-day clinical evaluation is obviously incomplete and too often extremely detrimental when we apply speculative labels to human beings and write them in our records. Examine the family as well as the dysphasic person. The patient most often responds more freely at home among his cushions of maximal security. Much of what his family observes can help you far more than any test or, for that matter, any of the discussions in the pages of this text. Patients respond better and more freely when they are secure enough to relax than when they are under tension of our clinical domain.

We must bear in mind in evaluating dysphasic patients that they may have an extensive oral vocabulary coupled with a pretraumatic perfectionism. The latter may expand beyond control after their accident. These perfectionistic persons may be unable to tolerate any error in their utterances, and so they choose to remain totally silent. The more they are pressured the more determined they become to say nothing. However, once they are convinced that their conversant is not likely to interrupt or to correct their utterances, they may feel the permissiveness enough to initiate brief communications. The dysphasic patient is always very sensitive to judgmental responses from his clinician after he becomes able to trust him. He will then request assistance and rely on the clinician's assessment of his communicative adequacy.

A rather dramatic example of such a behavior was revealed by

Mr. *W*. He had a very mild paralysis of the right side of his body, and there was no obvious interference with the movement of the oral mechanism. Mr. *W*. had always been a rather quiet person and did most of his recreational activities in isolation. He had also tended to reject people who were careless with grammatical rules. When he spoke, his fellow workers and family members were acutely aware of the outstanding clarity of his thought processes. Immediately after his neurological assault, he attempted to converse, but within a week all speaking was terminated. He seemed to understand oral directions with accuracy and was showing a marked interest in the daily newspaper and the television programs. Nevertheless he continued to remain completely silent.

When Mr. *W*. was referred to a speech clinic, six months later, he was still nonconversant. He always carried a newspaper or a small monthly magazine. Eventually his clinician began to question him about various articles in the paper and the patient pointed to the specific answers in print. One day a particular news item seemed to concern him seriously, and he was asked to read the article aloud. Much to the surprise of his clinician he did so with complete accuracy and articulatory fluency, but even then he failed to follow through with any spontaneous discussion. During the days that followed, however, he gradually initiated some attempts to discuss newspaper articles. Fortunately the clinician was wise enough to listen. This quiet attentiveness lessened the threat of interruption and seemed to stimulate an increase in the patient's verbal outflow. Shortly thereafter Mr. *W*. began to discuss his fears of erroneous language usage. It became evident that the communication problem was not solely due to an organic loss of language controls but to the erosion of the patient's self-confidence. Actually, his language utterances were only mildly impaired when he was no longer threatened by interruptions from his clinician. At this point the communication problem became more clear, and appropriate retraining procedures became more productive. It was evident that familial counseling was again a major obligation if there was to be any carry-over of the patient's willingness to communicate outside of the clinical boundaries.

Most of us tend to camouflage our weaknesses. We often feel demoralized when our friends and family members fail to give us a chance to discuss our attitudes confidentially. Our dysphasic patients are also mature human beings and are most apt to behave as such if we provide some pathway to security.

In order to balance the scale of this diagnostic discussion it seems important to consider carefully another patient at the opposite end of the continuum. Mrs. *D.*, a 54-year-old housewife, had spent the vast majority of her time with the chores of her household tasks. For some time her husband had been chronically ill and required considerable attention. She managed to retain a limited contact with her church, but this was the extent of her social activities outside the home environment. Shortly after her husband began to recover a limited independence, Mrs. *D* suffered a cerebral hemorrhage. Not only did she experience a total flaccid paralysis to the right side of her body but she also suffered a complete absence of expressive language. She did not appear to understand even the simplest discussion of daily events. Some five months after the assault she regained sufficient muscle control for ambulation and self-care. Gradually some meaningless language utterances developed and one consistent phrase, "that darned old shoe," was uttered repeatedly during conversations with other people. She was examined at a center for communication disorders and failed to demonstrate any understanding of oral and written language. Standard tests of aphasia were apparently beyond her abilities, and so her clinic file was closed before any consultations with her husband were provided. She was then taken to a different center three weeks later, and there the examination results were encouraging enough to enroll her for assistance. Though the patient was seen twice a week, her husband was seen only for the initial interview. Within six weeks her biweekly contacts were terminated because she failed to demonstrate any progress.

The patient's physician was indeed conscientious and immediately referred her to a third center. It was observed there that Mr. *D* was also in need of intensive counseling both for his own personal problems and those concerning his wife's health and communication limitations. He was a poor listener, confused, and terribly anxious. His wife could no longer respond to his discussions concerning his own health. The added anxieties of his wife's condition spurred him to try an overabundance of useless language drills and excessive care for her slightest physical needs. In essence, she did not have much motivation for improvement under the tent of her husband's confusing overprotection. Actually, she had been rewarded for becoming a household "blob," and felt little need for any improvement.

In this case, it was not possible to evaluate the language abilities of Mrs. *D.* at all accurately until her husband demonstrated some control of his own self-concerns. He was referred to his physician for medical counseling. In the meantime, the speech pathologist informed Mrs. *D*'s neurologist of these circumstances and he in turn contacted Mr. *D.*, carefully explaining the necessity for increasing Mrs. *D*'s freedom from dependency needs. Upon the satisfactory completion of medical guidance the husband was enrolled for counseling in the speech clinic.

Soon there was considerable improvement in Mrs. *D*'s ability to produce meaningful single-word utterances. At this point, predictions for continued improvement became more realistic, and the evaluation results were far more accurate. Although this patient did not recover enough language to maneuver independently outside of her home, she did reacquire enough language to make her needs known, which in itself improved her management of the household. Furthermore, her husband demonstrated an obvious lessening of his anxieties concerning both himself and his wife. It is significant that the majority of her improvement did not occur until approximately one year after the date of her vascular accident.

The clinician's attitudes are vital in determining the progress and prognosis of his dysphasic patients. If few of the latter can completely regain all of their former language abilities, it is still clear that most of them can be helped. Goal setting must be realistic; both perfectionism and defeatism are to be avoided.

The dysphasic patient is often capable of sensing keenly our discouragement over his problems. If you have little faith or hope there is little, if any, chance that you can get a realistic evaluation. Therefore, when you recognize that your clinical attitudes cannot be altered, refer the patient elsewhere but take care to avoid an expression of your own negativism. Simply request a consultation. If you are unable to modify your own attitudes, also make the transfer a permanent one. None of us has the ability to maintain perfection in all of our interpersonal relationships—but we can be honest and therefore increase the chances for our client's recovery, if we recognize our own limitations. This kind of honesty is essential.

I must remind you again that at one time or another, a significant number of patients express a death wish. When a patient says he wants to die, he means it. No language drill will lessen that desire; it may only increase it. Hear him out. The freedom to express such negative feelings often relieves the urge to escape his difficulties. Furthermore an astounding amount of language facility may be revealed. Be sure that you relay such information to your colleagues in psychiatry. This kind of death chatter is serious, and we speech clinicians are not the ones to accept the responsibility for relieving such dangerous attitudes.

It is probably clear by now that this author does not think there is one exclusive kind of language deterioration in dysphasia. Com-

12   In this introductory text we are avoiding the ordinary terminology used
to describe dysphasic behavior. We feel that most of the labels are im-
precise and, in general, more harmful than useful. However, for students
who wish to explore this terminology we can refer them to the references by Wepman (23) and Eisenson (5).

munication abilities depend on the coordination of a host of varied
neurological pathways within the brain. The slightest short circuit
in this patterning can alter the accuracy of understanding even the
simplest language; can disorder the emission of meaningful verbalizations; disturb emotionality; disrupt the stability of the self-concept;
and interfere with interpretation of the behavioral acts observed in
other people. It seems that Hughlings Jackson (1888) was indeed a
most insightful person. He was convinced that extensive observations
must first be accomplished before *any* clinical generalizations could
be made and even then such conclusions should be readily alterable
as new facts appeared. Every clinician should become acquainted
with the varied types of tests that are currently available. They are
tools that we all must use—but with sensitivity and discrimination.
They tell us much but I would also insist that we must not base our
impressions solely on the isolated test behavior of our clients. We are

13   A brief review of diagnostic tests used traditionally with dysphasic
patients can be found in the reference by Darley (4).

terribly obligated to get careful evaluations of the familial anxieties,
rejections, overprotection, and reduced self-esteem. Any diagnostic
category for the patient must truly include the measure and treatment of familial reactions to the deficit.

If the patient is a resident of a community, some one or two
hundred miles removed from your center, at least arrange to have
two contacts within the one day period. See him first at 9:00 A.M.
and again at 2:00 P.M. Best yet, see him a third time at 4 P.M. Even
though he is being seen in a community removed from his home,
the moderately damaged person is likely to be more alert during the
early morning. By 2:00 P.M. increased fatigue in itself can lessen his
accuracy, and at 4:00 he may indeed be obviously troubled. At this
time he is not only very tired but also anxious to depart for home,
all of which weakens his intellectual and language controls. Even a
latent dysarthria may become more obvious when the damaged
neural pathways are fatigued. Meaningless language expressions are
increased, and the patient's ability to respond accurately to your

verbal directions is also disturbed. Many utterances become increasingly garbled with tongue tremors that result from fatigue and increased depressive anxiety. Avoid these limited examinations if at all possible. The diagnostic examination of a dysphasic patient should be in the form of a broad longitudinal investigation.

Administrative Classifications

Three basic classifications seem necessary for the purpose of professional communication and relative orderliness of written records. These profiles are as follows: *Moderate Dysphasia; Severe Dysphasia;*

14   Compare this author's classification of severity with that used by
      Schuell (17).

and *Aphasia*. Some writers include in their classification a variety they term *Mild or Simple Aphasia*. It is this writer's belief based on long and personal experience that such a term is nonsensical. We shall begin therefore by describing moderate dysphasia.

Moderate Dysphasia

For the most part, the patients falling into this category will likely be successful in completing the majority of items on any standardized test for aphasia. Herein lies the greatest possibility for professional error, particularly if the evaluative impression is based solely on the test. When reactive speech is adequate during an initial evaluative appointment, detrimental conclusions are too often forthcoming from the examiner.

In some instances, transient cortical imperceptions occur. Sometimes it is impossible for these patients to understand your utterances at certain moments or to formulate their thoughts, even though the majority of time they seem to speak and to comprehend with apparent ease. Brief moments of bewilderment and anxiety are often the only cues to weakened perception. Moreover, in moderate dysphasia, if the patient fails a test because he cannot understand it at that particular moment, it does not mean that a similar failure will occur on the following day. Similarly transient imperceptions or difficulties in handling language can elude your attention if, on the day you see the patient, all is in relative order.

Articulation errors are particularly noticeable during the early weeks that follow the onset of brain damage. In some patients, this difficulty persists despite relative recovery of language and motor functions. Sluggishness of articulation is increased as both the length and speed of utterances increase. The most obvious difficulty occurs on the sibilant sounds, followed by distortions of the stop plosives. The absence of velar plosives indicates a greater severity.

I like to interpret this behavior as realistically as possible. We have no current means for assessing or accurately measuring neurological fatigue; nor can we estimate with any absoluteness a patient's ability to accurately judge his own articulatory clarity. Our major concern is most often that of his language efficiency. To both the patient and the clinician nothing else may matter for a long, long time. But we must recognize that the patient's nervous system is often incapable of combatting even the slightest fatigue. With fatigue, any kind of articulatory utterance may be a major accomplishment. Indeed we rarely find a patient who is highly concerned about his articulation errors. But he knows what counts the most in successful communication and therefore he concentrates on the language he utters, regardless of his articulatory garbling. As youngsters, our own speech development began in the same way. Surely we can understand the patient's lack of concern if the speech sounds sluggish and distorted but the meaning comes through. We are obligated to be as insightful as our parents were and recognize the patient's errors but be willing to untangle them. It is wise to record the dysarthric errors, but you should not give them too much value. Regardless of what you may try to do about the dysarthria, success may not come because of permanent damage, but you can't be sure at the outset. Spontaneous recovery does occur and it is more likely to if anxieties from unnecessary clinical pressures are removed.

Patients with *moderate dysphasia* often show erratic difficulties in finding some of the words they need. Even synonymous utterances are at times impossible for them. Mispronunciations occur inconsistently. Most utterances are appropriate, but during the course of conversation variances in syllabic stress occur, syllables may be inverted, and complex patterns of identical speech sounds may be impossible to utter when they occur a second time in the same phrase. When asked where he lives, he may respond as follows: "I live on the east—no—the south—no—the west side, yes the *west* side on Perry Street—no—on—you know—on Peach Street—yes, on Peach Street over in—no—*here,* in town." He may call his *sister* his *mother* and his *wife* his *sister.* The longer the language units become, the more he may reveal errors in his utterances. Concentration, even in moderate dysphasia, is indeed limited, so the examination should be short.

Most of our tests fortunately demand little abstraction beyond very simple levels, and these patients often perform these meager tasks successfully.

15   For another discussion of how to get your dysphasic patient to begin speaking, see the reference by Keenan (9).

A twenty-four-year-old male had been in an auto accident and had suffered damage to the left prefrontal area of the brain. There were no apparent symptoms of paralysis and no *obvious* signs of reduced controls in language. He complained of a problem but could not be specific or give a descriptive account of his difficulties. His emotions were exaggerated; he was either too gleeful or too tearful. But the longer he conversed the more he erred in expression. Most persons would not have known he had dysphasia. Only he knew the occasional lapses of continuity because they were not readily detectable, but he knew them well—and he was very concerned. His wife chuckled because she was unable to recognize the lack of continuity in his conversation, and the patient, of course, found her reaction insulting.

When the clinician opened a topic for discussion the patient immediately joined in and did his utmost to dominate the discussion. Each time the clinician interrupted the client's verbosity, even without changing the topic of conversation, the patient had great difficulty with the interchange. He not only had a temporary increase in dysarthria, but he also floundered in responding. He seemed to forget momentarily what he had been discussing. As this occurred, there was a shade of panic; his face became flushed and his irritability increased. His wife broke into the discussion and reprimanded him for his offensive emotional behavior. He, in turn, retorted with condemnation of both himself and his wife's "nosiness." Even though the clinician did his utmost to pursue the topic, the patient refused or was unable to respond through the "teary mist" of his profound frustration.

A new subject was brought up, and eventually the patient tried to join in, but this time his rambling seemed senseless despite a voluminous outflow of language. His wife remarked that this occurred often, but she thought it was due to his violent temper. "He can talk if he wants to!" she said. It was most apparent that his wife needed information, counsel, and insight. The stress induced by her misunderstanding released even more dysphasia as well as feelings of worthlessness and rejection. Most of all, his health was endangered, for peaks of anxiety tend to restrict the orifices of the blood vessels and increase the possibility of rupturing them. A medical re-referral was made in combination with a series of educational counseling appointments for his wife. The communicative problem was far from simple once the entire picture of the disruption was revealed. Interpersonal anxieties and conflicts can be dangerous in moderate dysphasia.

Many of these patients with moderate deficits in speech and language retain a relatively higher level of performance in reading activities than in speech. This, of course, does not mean that there is no reading problem, nor does it necessarily mean that they will recover their premorbid levels of ability. Most of the difficulty will be a result of shortened memory span or lack of interest in reading. It is particularly important to note that arithmetical and numerical improvements seem to accompany the recovery of language controls. Clinical efforts to help these patients with abstract numerical concepts are of no value unless the patient has adequate recovery in language. As a matter of fact, if the threat of failure in mathematical exercises is introduced before language manipulation is reasonably improved, even the least damaged person may experience further reductions in psychological and communicative adjustment. First things first, and language comes first! For this reason, if none other, it is wise to postpone retraining or assessment of mathematical abilities until after extensive speech and language recovery is obvious. In most instances, and if there is a real need for it, arithmetic ability will automatically return with language. We should make sure that the family constellation understands this danger, for unless they do, they can severely interfere with the recovery process. When a patient has need for written language and arithmetic concepts, he or she will let you know about it. When they are verbally capable of returning to their employment they will really benefit from such specific evaluations if they have a need for these abstract abilities. Don't let your evaluations create further hopelessness. Be realistic and be concerned; there is no room for routine clinical testing if thereby we increase the patient's problem.

Severe Dysphasia

Patients falling into this classification are characterized by an obvious reduction in vocabulary usage in all language modalities. Their utterances are telegraphic, and their receptive abilities may be equally damaged and foreshortened. Their abstract understandings are very difficult to measure. However, these people do have some

mild days during which their utterances are obviously more complete. It has been observed that the over-all energies are also
heightened at these times: the patients are eating better; they are
more likely to recognize even subtle good humor; they respond
better to making and receiving visits. In general, everything they do
is more normal during these rare but better periods. You can imagine
the negative impact of a sudden return to confusion, desolation, and
restricted communication during the bad days. Not only is there an
organic change to which the patient must adjust, but there is also
the negative psychological impact of felt regression.

This particular group of severely dysphasic patients have a living
pattern quite different from normal. Most of them have rare occurrences of energetic alertness, of being able to respond symbolically.
But they do have some good days, and it is our responsibility to detect
them before recording a label in the clinical records. There is a vast
difference between *severe dysphasia* and *aphasia*. A clinical folder is
so terribly permanent; be careful to delete the possibility of biasing
later clinicians when the patient moves on to other clinical domains
or when you seek new employment.

Sensorimotor impairments seem to dominate the severely dysphasic
patients. The absence of sensation is indeed a major problem when
one considers the fine and rapid adjustments necessary for spoken
language. This absence of sensation alone can distract the patient's
attention from what other people are saying and makes it difficult
for him to pay attention to his own formulations. This is particularly
true during the many months immediately following the accident
and is often erroneously classified as a cortical language reduction.
Sometimes the apparent lack of expressive ability is an intentional
avoidance of biting the tongue and cheek.

I experienced this kind of a problem in motor interference and
sensory distraction for three years after my accident. I still bite my
tongue or cheek occasionally when I'm tired, even though much
sensory recovery is evident. In one sense the problem is worse now
because the stimulus of returning pain has added further distraction
to expression or reception. Listeners often interpret this to be a
recurrence of my language deficit, and if this helps them to accept
me, I worry not. But in the beginning it was terribly disturbing. Any
attempt to expand my utterances only increased the swelling of my
right cheek and tongue. This, of course, increased dysarthria to the
point of total gibberish. It was safer to be telegraphic. Then at least
others responded to my utterances and lessened their offensive sym-

pathy. Bear this in mind as you contact your patients. Get and retain the concept of *sempathy* and dry your muddy ruts of tearful pity if you want to help.

Motor involvements in the severe dysphasic show a true consistency of articulatory errors. The sounds that require the most precision of movements are most apt to be defective. Polysyllabic words are less intelligible because they require a rapidity of soft tissue adjustments. Furthermore, with a reduction of sensation, sounds with similar articulatory loci are more apt to be confused or distorted. There is little the patient can do to rectify these errors without basic neurological recovery. Initially he is as helpless as you would be if you were a fullback on a professional football team.

A significant number of severe patients may appear to have lost all functional speech, and they may also refuse to attempt any imitation of their clinician's utterances. This behavior gives an impression of total aphasia when actually they are only fearful of hearing their own verbal slush or gibberish. Once they become acquainted with the clinician and feel secure in the clinical environment, they are more likely to make attempts at language expression that may surprise you. As may be surmised, language then becomes much improved, particularly when topics do not require lengthy responses. Such improvement is more apt to occur in a clinical living room that has no implication of formal testing. In relaxed interaction, self-attention is lessened, and articulatory deficits become less obvious to the speakers. When these severely impaired patients enjoy conversational activities even the spasticity decreases, and the amount of dysarthria is lessened. We must constantly seek to remove stress and threat. Even the slightest threat to a damaged ego may create a total withdrawal from social interaction, and silence is often the last remnant of control over interpersonal contacts. The more anxious these patients become, the more their thought processes shrivel. Clinicians must not make them worse than they have to be.

It is unfortunate but true that many patients are erroneously classified as severe aphasics when their major problem is that of paralysis of the oral structures. They behave as aphasics because they find little reason to elicit the conversation of others when their own articulatory abilities are absent. Furthermore, they avoid social contact as much as possible in an effort to lessen the repeated traumas of severe embarrassment. Even when there is only a moderate paralysis of the dominant hand, their written script is rarely legible, which also contributes to a false impression of agraphic aphasia. Damage to the brain limits their energies as well as their memories and contributes to emotional defeat. A false impression of severe receptive damage when all that is wrong is paralysis can have a profound effect on the patient. We must continuously examine our own observations and assumptions lest we falsely presume that irreparable language loss exists when this is not the case. The patient always needs the benefit of the clinician's self-doubt.

Even though I have reason to avoid such diagnostic errors, they have occurred in my own casework during periods of careless laxity. Fortunately, I have rigidly insisted on repeated visits when I work with dysphasic patients and have often had to alter my misdiagnosis. One patient in particular comes to mind in this discussion. A 50-year-old housewife was first seen in a hospital two weeks after her cerebral accident. There was no observable paralysis in her leg and arm; there was a slight drooping of the right face; but a reasonable control of her gross tongue and mouth movements was apparent. Vocalizations were barely audible and indeed meaningless. Obvious intellectual confusions and limited memory further lessened the accuracy of my prediction of possible recovery of language function. Such a qualification was recorded in the initial report. She was discharged from the hospital to her home, which was 100 miles from the clinical center. No help was available to her there. The patient traveled to the clinic every two weeks over a three-month period. Despite the careful cooperation of her family group, nothing they did seemed to alter the complete lack of language expression and understanding. As a matter of fact, she seemed to be regressing even in her physical responses to the utterances of others. Spontaneous recovery seemed nonexistent. I consulted with her neurologist and my clinic's psychologist, each of whom concluded that the neurological language and intellectual controls were indeed completely destroyed. She seemed to be totally aphasic.

I had the dubious honor of relaying these impressions to her family. Fortunately, they had more courage than I. They told me that if I would agree to see her on a daily basis they would mortgage their home to acquire funds for residence in the clinical community. This, of course, stemmed from my prior complaints that limited contact with the patient was never to be trusted, and though I was loathe to have them make the financial sacrifice, I had no choice but to agree with their proposition.

Shortly after their move the patient seemed suddenly to come to life and began to babble attempted imitations of my utterances. She even chuckled at my humor and accurately followed verbal instructions even though they were abstract and unaccompanied by gestures.

She agreed to a psychological re-evaluation, and the results of the performance tests were high normal. Within three weeks her articulation improved enough for any person to understand her individual words. In due time phrases were formulated and when she was dismissed eight months later, oral communication was more than adequate for pleasant social survival. The only real dysphasia ever exhibited was that in expressing proper names, and even this deficit decreased before she left the clinic. Some dysarthria persisted, particularly during periods of physical fatigue, but she managed to slow down her utterances sufficiently to retain reasonable clarity. Such experiences prove that our professional labels can be terribly blinding. What might have happened to this patient had her family accepted our speculative and erroneous assumptions?

16   Some of the factors to be considered in determining a prognosis of language recovery are given in the reference by Eisenson (7).

Imagine what an experience in abstract arithmetic testing can do to encourage troubled silence and how total self-condemnation can increase following failures in the management of written script during testing. When the dominant side of the body is damaged and visual competency impaired, writing becomes an incredibly difficult task. We already know that in the dysphasic patient these abilities are likely to be reduced. Why then must we hurt the patient as a person? The total problem, not an isolated function, must always be confronted. In these patients the verbal retention span is short enough without being traumatized by trying to cope with abstract numbers or written and printed words. It may be many months, in fact even a matter of years, before either the need or the ability to cope with these more abstract activities returns. Many horrible things have been done to patients in the name of clinical diagnosis.

Perhaps the most profound example of the preceding discussion can best be demonstrated through a discussion of another personal experience. This concerns the writing of this text, which as you may guess has indeed been discouraging but in the end a rewarding experience. Approximately five years after my cerebral embolism I was invited to prepare this manuscript so that my personal experience compiled with my professional training might make a real contribution to the understanding of dysphasia. Both Dr. Van Riper and the editorial staff of Prentice-Hall were convinced that I was again capable of managing the written word. I could converse well enough, my spirits were high, and even I felt that I had come far from the rugged pits of disparaging failure. But the ugly heads of reduced ability to handle abstractions, limited recall, and shortened memory, marred my manuscript. I was shocked beyond words when I reread my pages after they had cooled off in my desk drawer. You can perhaps imagine how the old depression again floated to the surface of my psychological existence.

My first thought was a memory of the written chores in which I had failed so miserably during the first year after my assault. I rapidly convinced myself that I was still in that darkened chasm. For a time, no one could change my mind. If only I had not been tested and confronted with this loss in the ability to formulate my thoughts in writing five years before, it is very likely that this new evidence of my impairment would not have been nearly so upsetting. It would have disturbed me, yes, but the negative identification with my initial defunctness would not have added depth to that depression. I am certain that I, like many other patients with whom I've since had contact, would have considered this present difficulty in writing as mainly a result of lack of practice.

In my depression I threw the script away, called my colleague, and volunteered to withdraw from the ugly task. Through his kind offer to help me start again and through his profound and insightful acceptance of my emoting blubber, I again raised my faltering pen. Traumas were indeed numerous during the first half of these latter five years. At times I talked as badly as I had been writing. Weeks and even months of withdrawal from the task were imperative, not only for my benefit but to relieve students, friends, and family members from my intense anxieties. Fortunately my editor understood completely.

The latter half of this treatise has been most pleasurable because I seem to have at last recovered a great deal of my former ability. I have not studied the grammar books. They only interfered with my self-confidence and helped to retard even the slightest improvement. I talked what I had to say over and over, recorded what I was saying, listened with a critical ear, and only then proceeded to write my thoughts. In due time I discarded the recorder and just proceeded to write and write. At last I had a need to spell, write, and punctuate. I'm relatively certain that it could not have occurred sooner because my cortical controls had to be established first, regardless of any functional motivation; but *both* had to occur before any progress was forthcoming. It has been a *ten*-year battle, not a three-month or even a three-year process, and first came my oral language controls. Without them any script would have been dissipated in my damp well of written oblivion.

Most assuredly the course of this disease is often unpredictable. This is particularly true of emotional stability. We must continuously bear in mind that depression is an ever-present threat to these patients. If the patient cannot talk clearly and clarify his feelings we must then see him often enough to acquire some understanding of his physical gestures and facial expressions. These form a major vehicle for communication when oral utterance is limited. Psychiatrists frequently advise us to encourage all means of emotional expression and thus to assist the patient to lessen morbid tension. We must be as permissive and supportive as possible and share our observations with such consultants. They can help us greatly. A patient who was obviously stable before his accident must be aided to reacquire enough confidence to permit realistic adjustments first. From this point on, his management of language will become more evident, and we will then be able to evaluate his possible potential more realistically. What we need is not diagnostic examinations but *diagnostic therapy,* and we need time and understanding.

Very few of these patients with severe dysphasia are willing to initiate any written script until after maximal recovery in oral expression is obtained. They may appear to cooperate under stress because survival in the clinic is simpler that way, but carry-over to outside activities is usually nil, and discouragement predominates. This we do not need during evaluative procedures. Wait until the appropriate time arrives during the retraining process and be sure that each patient truly has a need for script and math before submitting him to your abstract demands.

For the most part, these patients make some responses through gestures and facial expressions. Though they may be unable to *volunteer* a meaningful utterance, they can often repeat the single word expressions of their clinicians. In some instances these individuals can only imitate your facial movements, that is, opening and closing the mouth, pursing the lips, extending the tongue and other similar maneuvers. In order to estimate their ability to understand your utterances without a visual stimulus from you, simply *ask* them to do these things. If they repeatedly fail, give them an occasional example, always being sure their egos are protected. Many times an extreme lack of self-confidence can be misinterpreted to mean a total deficit in understanding. When a patient is unable to tolerate variances in his performance he may resist any attempt to follow through until he is sure that your reactions are not threatening. As clinicians we need to remind ourselves continually that our patients are truly adults. They have been competent social beings; this above all else they have not forgotten. Anxieties are exaggerated, and security is terribly thwarted when they are treated patronizingly. They are not children. We must avoid the introduction of new and more complicated tasks until the patient has achieved some success with those on the simpler levels, but we must always remember that they are adults.

It takes real clinical skill to introduce requests for the imitation of simple and automatic expressions, without hurting their pride. Ask the patient to vocalize not alone but *with you*—a groan, a sigh, or a chuckle. If he shows some ability to do some of these things on his own volition, try some humming, then follow with some simple songs that he enjoyed in the past. Words may then be forthcoming with little effort, and this may encourage him to try conversant utterances at a later time. Follow this with an example of your counting and ask him *to join you* in the activity when you start over. Let him keep on counting as far as he feels able to do so. The same procedure can be used for the days of the week. At this point, excuse yourself from the room to make a phone call or see a colleague. Suggest to him that he continue doing some of these things until you return. If you have an intercommunication system, turn it on before you depart. Better yet, if you have a closed circuit TV or a one-way mirror, watch him to see if he can make repetitive attempts in isolation. He may surprise you.

At this point it seems wise to avoid telling the family anything about this diagnostic activity. Most family groups will be so pleased with any utterance that they may overstimulate and therefore demoralize such a patient beyond endurance. We too must be careful to avoid such pressures. The main thing is to help him get his oral structures in action, to get vocalization and some success in saying something that sounded familiar. Neither what he says nor how he says it matters at this point. The simple fact that he has vocalized something, anything, may encourage him to try again and again.

Never be dishonest with the patient. If on Monday his isolated productions were relatively articulate, reward him accordingly. But, if on Thursday his verbal recall is sparse and articulation is more sluggish, avoid undue approval for his performance. He will be aware of the difference, and his consequent anxiety will be severe enough without having to listen to the clinician's "stupid praise" for nonexistent success. When a professional person treats him like a baby, the dysphasic patient's confidence in his clinician's judgment is jeopardized. When this occurs, the drive for continuing attempts is lessened and too often lost. Casually comment on the successes and most importantly acknowledge an inadequate performance by simply having him try it again. If it improves, the patient will probably recognize it and will then benefit from your honest reinforcement. Let him know that such variability in performance is common among the other patients, that this is a normal process in recovery of language controls. His feeling of isolation may then be lessened and repeated attempts more apt to be forthcoming.

Be sure that requests for verbal utterances are realistic. True, one of the first things we learned in school was the alphabet. But must we always ask a dysphasic person to labor so hard to get it right? The vast majority of our population seldom needs to utter the entire alphabet after departing from first grade, and your patient is not a first grader. The ability to recite by rote a silly alphabet may not be as automatic as one might suspect, particularly for individuals who were not involved with desk work. And certainly the failure to do so can traumatize the patient. Besides, is the alphabet truly an expression of language? How concrete is it? What real reward comes to the patient who is finally, after long labor and many failures, able to manage uttering the isolated and meaningless sounds so far removed from the basic needs of his social survival? These questions also apply to naming the 50 states and even the streets of his surrounding neighborhood. How many persons with dysphasia have been bedeviled by such tasks! *Be realistic with your expectations of the patient's performance and make sure you are capable of doing the things that you ask your patient to do.* People who have *severe dysphasia* can see no need for such utterances. Neither can you unless you need psychiatric help.

I stress this point as I recall the levels of demoralization experienced during the early weeks that followed my stroke. Friends and colleagues were truly doing their utmost to help me, but I rejected most of their drills and ultimately refused to attempt conversational activities with many persons. It was obvious, though evidently only to me, that the more they pushed me to verbalize, the less they could understand my utterances. The old vicious cycle raised its ugly head. The harder I tried to be articulate and to improve my language, the more I failed, and the more I failed, the less I cared about anything. My best protection from their pressures was that of utter silence. Even this behavior did little to protect my ego when I overheard their incredibly stupid comments about my withdrawal behavior. Their assumption of progressive intellectual regression almost convinced me that it was true. No one, other than my wife, seemed to recognize the intense emotional trauma as a possible reason for my lack of communication. Colleagues were as guilty of these practices as I had been before my own accident. I truly felt sorry for the patients who had suffered from my past stupidity. Perhaps my long labors on this book will make amends.

Occasionally it is wise to explain and to make apologies for requesting simple tasks of expressive performance. Show that you respect your patient and his potential. Keep the concrete activities realistically alive as you increase the amount of verbalization required. Cast the printed page aside; utilize existing objects and structures for language stimuli. It may seem terribly slow to operate this way, but the ceiling of abstraction depends wholly on a solid foundation of concreteness.

Very few patients are willing to hear their own futile and defective expressions over a lengthy period of time. They will soon avoid all attempts to respond if their conversants persistently push them down the monotonous trail of idle expression. It is possible for some patients to utter meaningful words if allowed to repeat phrases in unison with the examiner. For example, point to the door and say, "I open the door," and do so. Do this several times and then ask the patient to join you in unison, both in speech and activity. Speak slowly, give him a chance to make adjustments for his paralyzed musculature, *and wait!* After two or three trials in unison, reduce your phonation or pantomime the words with no voice so he can hear what he can do by himself. If he is able to produce it as he watches you, mouth the words. Lastly, ask him to say the meaningful sentence by himself with no auditory or demonstrable assistance from you during his utterance. If each step is successful, then of course, predictions for eventual success are indeed encouraging, provided that neither the patient nor his clinician become overanxious for rapid progress.

What about those clients who cannot successfully complete all these communicative steps? Explore the ability to simply fill in statements accompanied by your actions. Walk to the door, open or close it, repeat the word *door* several times, have him try it in unison and then in isolation. Even though his utterance may not be intelligible, if he vocalizes *something* you at least know that he is still aware of the necessity for language, has a drive for expression, and is thus not totally unaware of the need for spoken language. Do the same thing with other structures such as *wall, window, floor, light, chair, book, telephone, pencil, paper,* and *table.* Avoid using pictures. Drawings are even more difficult for the severely dysphasic person. Use the things that the patient can touch and manipulate and explore. It is not uncommon for a woman to be *unable* to say "purse" when it is pictured, but as she holds or opens her own purse the word often slips out with little effort.

Some patients can respond well to your starter phrases and actions that introduce the words to be elicited. Rather than quietly pointing to the window, say, "We look out of the _____," and await the patient's attempt to complete the statement, but always finish it if he does not. He may join you. Many other similar statements may be used, that is, with a doorkey in hand say, "I lock the door with a _____(key)." Point to the bookcase, "We read _____(books)"; as you point to your chair say the phrase, "I sit on a _____(chair)"; and pick up the phone saying, "I talk on the _____(phone)." Constantly strive to maintain your ingenuity in devising appropriate meaningful activities and utterances. It is also wise at times to verbalize what the patient is doing, perceiving, or feeling—and always in simple language.

This discussion brings to mind a specific patient who failed to follow through on every procedure that we used to stimulate voluntary vocal responses. On her eighth visit, it was decided that evaluative appointments should be terminated. I suggested to her that we stop because another person was due to see me and said in closing, "I'll see you." She blurted out the word "tomorrow." Immediately I tried other leading phrases, and each time she accurately supplied the missing words, each of which we had previously attempted in isolation. Needless to say, clinical appointments were continued. In a very few weeks she began to utter the carrier phrases in combination with the key words. Conversations became meaningfully enjoyable outside of the clinical confines, and she gradually returned to her former shopping and family routines with adequacy.

17   A fascinating account of a dysphasic patient's self-therapy will be found in the reference by Bixby (1).

Each of us is ego-centered, brain-damaged or not, and we resist being manipulated. Unfortunately, this resistance is something we seldom recognize in ourselves or even in those persons who seek our guidance. Too often we talk to our dysphasic patients as though they were manikins under our control and in our power. Many of the dysphasic patient's expressions are like tiny fragile ropes on which the patient tugs restlessly in an heroic effort to pull the wavering words back for useful emission so he can assert himself and maintain his integrity. If you listen with kind attentiveness and respect, at least the danger of your rude interruption, with its implication of your power over him, is quelled. This gives him more freedom for communicative experimentation. Let him have the time and opportunity to reconstruct the damaged links of personal expression. Don't strain them before the solder is cool enough to withstand your clinical tug. Cast aside practices of interrogation and demands that you have been conditioned to endure. Final oral examinations are ridiculous enough in the academic world. We need no oral examinations in dysphasic therapy.

It is sometimes helpful to start a discussion by some self-directed talk or anecdotes. They may open up pathways of self-thought in the patient. Much of what you have experienced in the past is markedly similar to that which your listener knows well. You each have a hometown, have attended schools, had favorite teachers, brothers, sisters, and the like. In turn, ask the patient about such things and then be casually attentive to that which he utters. There is no hurry; help him disregard the pressure of time. Describe your abode and let him know you also have an interest in his home. Again, give him plenty of time to attempt its description. Always look for progress. Determine the completeness of his utterances. Are they solely an enumeration of objects or is there now a mixture of both isolated words and short phrases? Are his ideas expressed more meaningfully? How long can he continue before welcoming a cessation of your verbal interaction?

As time goes on, personal interrelationships will more than likely become warmer and thus relax the tension of strangeness and confusion. It takes time for the clinician to successfully adapt his own speech to the receptive level of his client, to learn the patient's language and limitations. The patient needs time and so does the clinician. Both must have it.

This casual kind of verbal activity can give us an estimate not only of the patient's ability to manage language, but also of the extent of his memory span. *If the latter is terribly short, then enrollment for language retraining will likely be futile until after it is increased.* Memory span almost wholly depends on improvements in the cortical blood supply, in relative freedom from emotional upset, and maximal patience on the part of those persons with whom the patient resides. There is but little we can do through demand or pressure. Should we pressure him too early or too much, we will only make his refusals to try permanent. Even after cortical controls become evident, he may not be able to overcome the effects of his past failures.

Avoid the printed page in your clinical interactions with most patients. Even pictures are abstract and have but one dimension; they are not *things*. We must remember that what we are after is to improve the basic level of understanding what is being said and spoken. His ability to interpret printed matter is much less vital. First things first!

Nothing can be so vital as the attitude of the clinician. If it is essentially negative the patient stands little chance for change or growth. This is particularly true if we blindly assume that reception is seriously impaired. Conversely, if he appears to be listening attentively it does not necessarily mean that he is absorbing the meaning of your utterances. You too can "fake it" when you are entangled in the vines of verbal confusion. He will stop pretending if he feels you are competent and understand him.

Aphasia

Cold basic facts are indeed difficult for even professional personnel to accept readily. But we are assuredly obligated to be completely honest with the families of our patients even though what we have to tell them may be unpleasant and negative. There are many brain-damaged people who will never be able to show improvement in language despite long and intensive help from the most skilled clinicians. Many of these patients with a poor prognosis never seem to become discouraged. This in itself is often an indication of severe damage to the intellectual processes. It may reflect a lack of realistic memory span, or simply the desire to have something other to do than just "hang around the house." Many patients are too pleasant. They agree with anything and everybody and joyously babble non-sensical responses. They are overly cooperative. Much of their behavior is simply a mirror-like reflection of the behavior in other persons. If the clinician or member of the family is sad, they too assume a similar facial expression. When joyousness reigns, the patient's response is also amiable. Such behavior is terribly misleading because it falsely signifies an abstract understanding of events and discussions. Frequent appointments are indeed crucial because nearly all patients behave this way at times, particularly if they suffer from epilepsy or frequent periods of extreme fatigue. Many are also subjected to such intensive pressures for speech in the home environment that if they babble something, anything, it reduces the demands of the family group. Such instances must be determined before we draw the final conclusion that profound organic damage makes the prognosis very poor.

Mr. *F.* had suffered a cerebral hemorrhage approximately sixteen months before he was taken to a language clinician for assistance.

By this time there was very slight evidence of right body dysfunction, but as yet he had not been able to utter any meaningful language. As a matter of fact, his only expressions were "la-la," "ee-ee," and "oo-oo." He had not been seen by a neurologist since his dismissal from the hospital six weeks after his hemorrhage. Therefore, he was referred immediately to the consulting neurologist who reported that there was a slight sensory deficit in the right face and tongue, very minimal paralysis in the right body, relatively normal readings on the EEG, and no apparent reductions in visual acuity. His hearing (pure-tone) seemed to be within normal limits for all frequencies, and there was no evidence of an otological dysfunction. Furthermore, there had never been any symptoms of epilepsy, nor was there reason to believe that there was any current difficulty. The entire medical picture was indeed a positive one for survival, and there was no reason to doubt some recovery of language use.

As might be expected, Mrs. *F.* revealed increased anxiety. Their four youngsters were attending a university, which, of course, created a marked financial burden. Mr. *F.* had graduated *cum laude,* and this fact alone made it difficult for her to be casual in accepting his mental deterioration. She had been dependent on him for nearly all the major familial decisions regarding monetary matters, as well as most social activities. Her self-rejections seemed to dominate all familial attitudes. Psychological counseling was necessary to relieve her pangs of guilt, which with time provided more freedom for her supportive relationships with her husband.

The language clinician cautioned the family to realistically control their expectations regarding the patient's social readjustments. Mr. *F.* was seen twice a day for a three-week period before his wife was permitted to join the sessions. Concurrently, she was being seen each day by the psychologist, and it was determined that she could attend her husband's clinical sessions at the beginning of the third week because of obvious improvements in her self-attitudes.

During this period, there had been no progress whatsoever in her husband's language interaction with the clinician. Psychological examinations revealed excessive mental deterioration to the level of idiocy. His behavior was identical with that of a mongoloid. He was extremely affectionate with all persons; emotional responses were identical reflections of those exhibited by the examiner, and there was no evidence of useful memory for any activity beyond nutrition. When the clinician smiled, Mr. *F.* mirrored the expression. If the clinician frowned or looked sad, the patient's face altered accordingly, regardless of the topic of conversation. The clinician could berate the patient furiously, but as long as he smiled and laughed while doing so, Mr. *F.* joined in. When humor was expressed with a sad facial countenance, the patient imitated to the point of tears.

Comprehension was obviously limited for body parts: arm, eye, leg, etc. Writing was absent although he had repeatedly been instructed to trace the script of simple and common words. Coins and monetary bills seemed to have no meaning, even when coffee was purchased at the neighboring snack shop. None of these failures altered his attempts at imitation nor did he lose his smiling affection for his wife and clinician.

Mrs. *F.* carefully continued to maintain stimulation in home activities throughout the following three weeks in combination with daily clinic visits. It became increasingly evident to her that little could be done to recover the almost complete loss of former aptitudes; her husband was demented. Mr. *F.* was seen quarterly throughout the ensuing year and despite his wife's careful stimulus of language no changes became evident. He remained congenially affectionate despite his own sociointellectual vacuum. Throughout the following two years, other clinics were visited and each confirmed the same severity of damage. This act in itself was therapeutic for the family; they needed to feel that they were doing and had done their utmost to help their patient. This patient truly had aphasia.

There are varied degrees of this most severe disruption that I prefer to call *aphasia*. Some such persons are less aphasic than others, but none are able to reach the slightest level of psycholingual independence. They cannot retain recent memories, nor can they recall those existing before damage to their brains. There may be minute periods of apparent exhilaration, but these are short-lived and extremely rare. The plateaus are permanently consistent. The true aphasic is unable to respond appropriately to testing or diagnostic therapy. Even the emotionality seemingly remains consistent, and the most fortunate ones are those hebephrenic "happy ones" similar to the case we have just mentioned. The patients who are consistently irritable will be institutionalized. This, of course, is often necessary for the welfare of familial groups who, after all, must be helped to confront the necessity for institutionalization. They always need help in making the decision to confine their patients, and the speech clinician should solicit the assistance of personnel in related professions. The most important thing to know about an observation is that it must be made more than once, by more than one person, and by more than our one profession. Truth is not a private affair; it is founded on the open ledger of fact. It can be painful, yes, but clean operative honesty in such a decision is far superior to prejudice, hostility, or blatant deceit.

BASIC PRINCIPLES OF RECOVERY

Speech clinicians have much to learn after they receive their academic degrees. Even experienced clinicians must be continuously alert to the positive cues that arise from hour to hour that can continue to educate them. Our clients will be our best teachers if we are willing to display our receptiveness. Clinical techniques must always be adapted to each patient. With this in mind you may better understand why we have not included many specific procedures in this manuscript.

We are each endowed with an extensive number of individual experiences, many of which have little bearing on anyone other than ourselves. This is particularly true of brain-damaged adults. Our major purpose should simply be that of trying our utmost to increase each patient's language functioning to the best of his cortical ability, his individual needs, and for the benefit of those persons with whom he must survive. We must bear in mind that the clinician, the patient, and his family must explore, adapt, seek, and incorporate each little bit of individual progress. The basic grunts of vocal reaction, the gestures and facial expressions can become meaningfully supportive to the recovery of word usage. Our honesty in reaction is essential to the patient's progress; don't try to fool him into believing you understand what he means when you don't understand it. He will soon know you are bluffing and quickly withdraw and isolate himself from your clinical blunders. Instead, let him know that his attempts are unclear, tell him what you interpreted and give him a chance to try again. If after two or three times he fails to make his purpose clear, apologize for your inability to interpret his communicative acts and suggest that the topic be dropped for the moment. Then initiate a new topic for discussion, or a new activity. Casually guide his responses, help him to retain his meager drive to interact with you. The patient and you, his clinician, must work together, he guiding you as you also guide him.

When the patient's momentary level of success has been discovered, casually and carefully attempt to extend the achievement bit by bit and keep moving *with the patient.* If you get behind, you insult him and worse yet, if you are too far ahead, you demoralize him. Work with what he needs to work on. Help him (and his family) to live within his limitations so that he may recognize that he can survive in spite of most of his losses. When this revelation occurs, the patient will find more time to pay heed to his language problems. Even slight progress in daily living will encourage attempts at the socialization that after all is predominantly based on meaningful verbal interchange.

The most severe *dysphasics* (not the aphasics) have a storage of premorbid language that is relatively intact. Many of them can occasionally respond to your gesticulations with an appropriate utterance of words, phrases, and even sentences. Your own silence may be the first they have encountered since their accident; try it out—give them a chance to experiment. Many of them have much to say when their fear of interruption is minimized. They will then await your reaction to their successes, but be calm about them. The patients will be excited enough without an elaborate show from you. Remember that their stream of nervous impulses can easily short-circuit into uncontrolled emotion if they get too excited. A simple nod of your head combined with a facial expression of pleasure will let him know that you heard. His thought will then be more coherent and less apt to be interrupted, and he may be more able to finish his sentences than if you show undue surprise, pleasure, or enthusiasm. Don't forget your role. You are a clinician, not an elementary classroom teacher. A good clinician is there to stimulate attempts at utilizing language; to communicate with the patients; and above all to provide a good example of the ability to listen and to respond appropriately.

Most people talk too fast and say too much to dysphasic persons. Even we who are normal make occasional complaints about our friends' and associates' garrulity. Our dysphasic clients have frequent and repetitive lapses in understanding spoken words. The condition is worse when they are tired and have added aches and pains. Brain damage lessens attentiveness and reduces the ability to understand the words of others. Your oral utterances to them can sound like a foreign language, particularly in the absence of visual cues. Stay on a simple language level, incorporate objects that can be seen and actions that can be shared or imitated. Meaningful patterns of stimuli are profoundly important for preparation in condoning more abstract events. The words we use must be those that are utilized most often and most meaningfully. They must be reused time and again in order to stabilize the foundation for eventual abstract understanding, but formal drills are the province of the stupid clinician. The regaining of lost language will usually be very gradual, and it must be useful or it will never return.

Peculiarly, many of us seem to feel that increased vocal intensity aids communication with our more silent partners. Even people on vocal rest to assist the remediation of acute laryngeal infection complain that some friends seem compelled to shout at them. Imagine the continuous anxiety of the dysphasic when his family, friends and, worst of all, his varied clinicians react in the same manner. Nothing is more likely to decrease attentiveness or stir up negative aggression than this shouting. But very few of my professional acquaintances seemed able to vocalize naturally to me after my accident. Many incorporated infantile vocal inflections and even regressed to the level of sweet baby talk. This was bad enough with a normal loudness, but did they have to *shout* their baby talk at me? Most dysphasic patients have similar complaints.

Be sure that the clinical room is a quiet one. Eliminate as many auditory distractions as possible; keep the environment orderly; and converse naturally if you want to help your patients retain some confidence in themselves. If they are truly hard of hearing, then seek the assistance of colleagues in audiology and otology, but otherwise avoid any instrumental amplification. It can be overwhelming and terrifying to the patient's damaged ego. These people are slow of thinking and reacting, but few of them are hard of hearing. They have an *emotional-intellectual deafness,* so converse with them accordingly. Casually slow down your rate of utterance until you observe an increase in the rapidity of their responses. In due time most of them will regain some quickness in their understanding of your utterances and only when this occurs and not before, may you increase the amount and rate of your verbal outflow.

Let us say again that our major purpose is that of stimulating the patient to make attempts at oral responses. Even though the response may be jargonish, if he is trying, and is appropriately rewarded for his attempts, positive results will tend to ensue. Be sure the family is aware of this need for reinforcement, but help them to maintain maximal objectivity. Let them know that the patient will likely be his own articulatory correctionist if he is allowed freedom for his exploratory trials.

Are There Any Specifics?

There certainly is one! We must do our utmost to change the negative attitudes that may be present in the household. This can be accomplished only through long, careful guidance and education for the major familial members. It must be assumed, of course, that we can help only those families who are willing and able to help themselves. If it is impossible to acquire cooperation, it is likely that the

18   An account of group counseling of families of dysphasic patients will be found in the reference by Turnbloom and Myers (20).

severely dysphasic patients will receive but very minimal benefit, if any, from our efforts. In such instances, we should do our utmost to find suitable placement in a convalescent home that has the services of a language clinician and careful interaction between related professional workers. Patients who are veterans can often be hospitalized in a V.A. center that is staffed to aid dysphasic persons. In this manner, the usual negativisms may be prevented or modified, and the basic recovery process is likely to be stimulated in such an environment. If you are compelled to continue treatment under adverse circumstances, set your personal goals accordingly. None of us are gods or even magicians, nor are our clients superhuman.

Sources of Language Stimulation

People with severe dysphasia can be easily distraught by printed material. Even clear photography lacks dimensions of depth. As we have said, pictures are flat, and the objects in them are reduced in size and shape; they are immobile and untouchable. Moreover, commercial sets of pictures contain objects that most people have rarely verbalized. Use real objects and common ones. Very few of our clients live in an elaborate setting; most of their household furnishings are simple in design. The same is true of clothing, automobiles, and even the shrubbery in their yards. Talk about the things and activities they know well.

As was stressed earlier, the patient will have a daily need for certain words to enhance his comfort and to fulfill his vital personal needs. If for no other reason, the clinical environment should be devoid of a desk and filing cabinets. These objects pose a threat to anyone because of their formality and negative identifications with past tensions. Our clients don't feel academic nor are they ready to incorporate a business-like attitude. A simply furnished living-room facility for language therapy is no more costly than the usual office furnishings of desks, chairs, and storage files.

Each person must be clothed, and most clothing must be selected for wear. Patients who are minimally mobile have to ask for many such articles, and they usually want to participate actively in decisions as to wearing apparel. A person's shirt, pants, socks, shoes, dress, sweater, purse, beads, earrings, and the like can provide meaningful stimuli for language. In due time colors can be added. Most of our patients are clothed all day; there is no need for pictures of these things. They are wearing them.

Living-room articles also provide a good source of stimulation—the davenport, chair, lamp, table, ashtray, radio, T.V., door, window, etc. Again, there is no need for pictures if the objects are continuously available for use. Real, concrete things possess dimensions and shadows. Permit my reiteration that we must begin at the level where the language has broken down, with the need to relate verbally to the real world about us. Be quiet long enough to give each patient a chance to reveal himself, to do some talking about this part of his real world, to handle the varied objects and clothing, and to experiment with attempts to verbalize in a clinical environment that is relatively free from negative threats to the ego.

Then, let us find an opportunity to go to another room of major interest—the kitchen. Both men and women have spent considerable time in it. The men have investigated the refrigerator, pantry, and cupboards for snacks. Some have even assisted their wives in mealtime activities or at least made their own breakfasts. Most of them continue to do so even after their accident. Remember that a hunger drive most often persists powerfully despite the extent of other behavioral losses. Women will often show an intense drive to return to the center of their major activities, the kitchen. In it they feel at home and secure. Much useful kitchen language may be expressed rather suddenly as they prowl through the cupboards, handle the familiar utensils, and examine the cartons and cans of foods. Both you and your fellow staff members should save such containers for use in the clinic. Open the bottom of the cans and cartons so they will retain an original appearance for storage in the clinic kitchen. Milk cartons, meat containers, and similar articles can be stored in the refrigerator. Visit major electrical and kitchen supply stores to explain your purpose. Most often a dealer will come through with a fine contribution of appliances taken in on a trade: kitchen sinks, refrigerators, kitchen stoves, and even dishwashers. Grocery stores have boxes for the display of varied foods, plastic fruits, meats, and vegetables. Take your clinical basket to them; they will be glad to fill it once they understand your purpose.

When the patient is able, make the clinical session one of simple mealtime preparations. Solicit the assistance of the patient's family group. Despite the fact that you may be a culinary expert, the stricken wife or mother needs stimulation that is commensurate with her former aptitudes. No one can know them better than the people she lives with. Through these activities they will come to know better how to stimulate the patient's outflow of language, if you have been careful to include them in your earlier clinical activities. Watch them from the observation room and always commend them before offering negative criticism. Keep in mind that dysphasic rehabilitation is a very frustrating though challenging task for all concerned. The family members in this situation are on display and initially they may be terribly self-conscious, so postpone any criticism until they become better adjusted. After due reward, they will likely solicit a description of their mistakes and consequently be more likely to rectify them. As you observe, record a summary of the activities that best seemed to stimulate the patient, then share your comments with the family and utilize it in your own follow-up contacts with the patient.

This kind of language stimulation is most certainly far superior to any commercial drill books or materials. None of us learned our own language in a threatening drill-filled classroom. Mom talked to us, played with us, and lovingly rewarded us for our progress. Remember your own development and be equally kind to your brain-damaged clients.

My professional friends and colleagues were somewhat distraught with my complete rejection of their commercial language drills and machines and books. I, too, was disturbed with my negative reactions, but I could not bear the insult of "grade school academics." Many words, phrases, and questions felt like the sharp edges of a razor blade immediately severing any desire to express anything but purple profanity. "Read this!" "Say this!" "Build a house!" they instructed me. First of all, I could care less about any kind of construction. I hated the thought of it. Secondly, I was paralyzed, and such a statement reminded me of my physical uselessness. "Build a house!" Thirdly, it was quite probable that I might never return to my role as the family wage-earner, and my home was then in danger of being lost to the finance company. "Build a house!" I had no use for such a statement. I would not put such a phrase in my mouth even if I could. It meant nothing to my social survival, and this was my primary concern. The blur of all these signal reactions erased the statement from my consciousness, and I responded with the usual "goddamnitall!" So—with a pat on my senseless knee my clinician offered another phrase, "knife and fork." I couldn't understand what was said nor could I follow his gesticulations, let alone interpret the picture of the articles he showed me. Knife and fork, indeed! I couldn't care less about naming these objects, even after I finally understood what he wanted. Who needed to talk about a knife and fork at such a time and in such a place? Besides, I was lucky to get even a *spoonful* of food to my mouth with my nondominant hand. I had no reason to concentrate on these words as I squirmed in my chair, trying desperately to postpone a trip to the toilet. We tried another phrase, "Drive the car." My cane was my car at the moment, and it was impossible for me to even think about successfully maneuvering my automobile through the congested streets. To me I was nothing but a blob to be transported by others. I couldn't even wash the windshield! There was no use for such a statement. I still had to go to the bathroom. Fortunately the language session terminated in time, but the word I needed the most was never introduced even when my clinician guided me down the hall to the toilet. As a matter of fact, that drillbook didn't even have a picture of a toilet. The next clinic session, I was asked "What do you drive?" A shrug of my shoulders was accurate in communicating my hopelessness of ever driving again, but the clinician insisted over and over again that I say "I drive a car." How much of my language inability and depression was organic? The weak enthusiasm for language management disappeared, but on we went with the same silly chores of that "damned drillbook," none of which had any connection with my real needs for survival or identity.

It was then that I determined someday to record my experiences in an effort to prevent such traumas for other patients. And oddly enough, I felt terribly guilty recalling my earlier professional stupidity with other dysphasics. I even felt compassion for those persons who were currently doing their utmost to assist me. But they were ignorant, and that ignorance was an evil that needed eradication.

The time to talk about any topic is when there is a *need* for such an utterance. Don't stimulate with the word *toilet* unless the patient is on the way to it. Talk about it then, and use it often in an effort to associate the numerous stimuli that are connected with such a trip. This of course can best be done at home by the persons with whom the patient lives. Above all, be certain that any language stimuli you use have a close connection with the life activities of your client. Choose and use those that are of maximal importance to the patient's needs and desires—not to yours. A significantly large percentage of patients who have experienced a recovery similar to mine have expressed their similar outrage regarding bookish clinical procedures and the use of drills.

Be Cautious With Reading Activities

Youngsters show little interest in reading the printed word before they have mastered their oral language fairly well. Even kindergarten activities have few reading drills. Most of the reading they do is picked up indirectly. We don't pressure them to read before they can talk. Those children who demonstrate an early ability to interpret some of the visual squiggles on the cans or cartons or street signs are indirectly reinforced casually by their parents. A good teacher is not a pusher; she is a supportive stimulator. When such children reveal an intellectual need for reading, the teacher helps. If help becomes pressurized, however, these youngsters quickly withdraw, and many of them show retarded reading skills in later years. Fear of failure can prevent progress. Surely we should recognize how this may also occur among our brain-damaged adults, particularly when they have not yet acquired a reasonable control of self-evaluation.

I have found it terribly important to wait until I have a certain indication of the patient's *need* for reading before using such activities. Usually this does not occur until after they are mobile and able to leave the home sanctuary. By this time there has usually been some evident recovery of reading street signs, labels on grocery containers, and newspaper headlines. Even those who have had a relatively extensive educational background find little need for reading until after they are neurologically able to withstand anxious fatigue. Medical clearance and common sense are of utmost importance before initiating the added stresses created by reading, and I speak of this from personal experience as well as from observations of other patients.

A vast number of our clients have had little need for reading once they departed from public school training. The truck-drivers, construction workers, hairdressers, and waitresses rarely did more than scan their daily newspapers. Illiterate people in the retirement years are rarely motivated to learn to read, but they manage to get along. If we are not sure that our patients have a desire to recover this ability, we may only increase their black crusts of demoralization on which they feed when alone. Reading too soon can halt conversational progress. This is not to say that there are no exceptions. Any rehabilitative program must be founded on the personal needs and abilities of each patient. There is no generalized program that is applicable to all patients, of course. Each one needs his own therapy design.

Most of my acquaintances in speech pathology are neither trained nor capable of managing a remedial reading program. I, for one, did not have sufficient study nor supervised clinical training in this activity. If we must move on to the teaching of reading, we who are untrained must refer our patients to appropriate reading centers, forwarding a detailed analysis of the patient's medical, psychological, and oral language abilities; only then carefully following the reading clinician's recommendations for specific techniques if they seem appropriate to our patient's needs.

Probably all speech pathologists would be very wise to acquire training in the management of reading problems. There is an extremely close relationship between oral and written language *after* these dysphasic patients have a reasonable control of their utterances. Each can help the other and thus solidify progress in over-all language controls. But again remember that each person must truly have a real need for reading before you try to help him regain it. We must always be careful to avoid the blind assumption that *all* clients will benefit from anything.

How Soon Should They Write?

There are four premises: (1) neurophysiological adjustments are indeed of prime importance; (2) intellectual and emotional abilities must be established; (3) there must be a strong personal need to write; (4) some control of oral language must have been achieved.

19   Some of the problems encountered in teaching the dysphasic patient
      to write are given in the reference by Smith (19).

Before delving into any consideration of methods for assisting the patient in writing—stop reading at this point. For the next eight hours or so record your lecture notes, button your clothing, feed yourself, and comb your hair with the sole use of your nondominant hand. Can you do it gracefully? Are you having trouble holding or guiding your pencil? Is there a distortion of letter forms? Are you writing complete sentences or is it easier to be telegraphic? How easy is it to spell the word you are writing? How soon did you decide that the whole silly experiment was futile and when did you drop the task?

A considerable number of patients are incapable of making adjustments to a shift in handedness for a matter of several months or even years. This is particularly true when they have little if any need for writing. Only a very small percentage of them do have an immediate desire, regardless of their pre-morbid needs. Oral expressions are enough trouble without incorporating the sweat-laden task of holding a pencil, let alone manipulating it through the horrible contortions of script on paper. You will discover that a number of patients are as hard-headed as I was; they are sure the paralyzed arm and hand will soon be normal. You'll not talk them out of it so don't waste their time. Besides, they may be right; so wait and see. Though very few do recover enough to use even a partially paralyzed hand for fine movements, some lucky ones do. Wouldn't you consider it a waste of time to train your nondominant hand and discover that the paralysis had regressed enough to use the dominant side? Do you write if you don't have to? Look at your lecture notes; they are scanty and incomplete, are they not? Answer this one: "Why do you put off writing those letters?" And you have no organic excuse, do you? Remember, the patient's language, thoughts, and memory are limited, and until each is under considerable control there is really little need for script. Regardless of what we may try to do, in teaching writing skills prior to language acquisition, progress will be nil. With recovery, this ability often returns, but it can be undetectable if an extreme sense of worthlessness persists. Far too many patients (and one is enough) fail to achieve recovery of usable language because of unwarranted clinical pressures.

During the later stages of oral language recovery, most patients will request assistance in writing. By this time, they will have done some experimenting on their own, particularly if they anticipate returning to former office work. Self-objectivity is usually enhanced, and they more easily recognize the futility of trying to use the paralyzed hand. Once they have found a personal need for writing they truly want some help and can profit from it. I have found that many patients can then train themselves by copying, and this is very good for their morale. Very few persons like to depend on others, and the majority of our dysphasic patients are honest enough to seek help when they need it. It will, of course, do no harm for you to volunteer assistance; it opens the door for them to accept it, or if they are reluctant, it permits them voluntarily to discuss it. Be careful not to push it. Always wait for them to agree that they need it.

I speak of this writing problem with a strong sense of obligation to fellow-patients. The vast majority react the same way that I did in that they (1) must have felt a need for writing, (2) that they could not be convinced that their paralysis would be relatively permanent, and (3) that without improved conversational ability, the writing chore is extremely demoralizing, let alone impossible. The only writing that I attempted for nearly a year after I returned to work was that of signing my name on dictated letters, checks, and grade cards. No one could convince me that my right hand was permanently disabled despite my prior clinical observations of many other brain-damaged clients. My emotional controls were weak and my intellectual disabilities interfered with reasonable foresight, let alone permitting the recall of my past clinical observations. If I, a fairly sophisticated speech pathologist, had such difficulty, it stands to reason that uninformed patients will surely be equally, if not more, resistant. Bear this in mind: be sure that they are ready, willing, and able to face their physical losses before attempting writing. It demands a great deal of abstract function. Unless there is a strong personal need for such training, over-all regression may occur.

You may question why I then attempted writing this text. For nearly three years, off and on, I simply used a dictaphone and then tried to edit my secretary's resulting typescript. I found I was getting nowhere and only adding confusion to existing confusion. There were strong temptations to terminate the chore but my unreasonable conscience would not allow it. At last I gave in, picked up my pen with my left hand, and suffered the miseries of south-paw script for weeks on end. It gradually became legible and relatively automatic but even now it is considerably slower than it had been with my right hand. I am certain, however, that had I not signed a contract with the publisher, my handwriting would still be nearly illegible. Enough said. Remember me as you approach your own clients; most of them will have had very little need for the pen.

We must also be sure to do our utmost to determine how well the patient can see before initiating any training in reading and writing. Let us take a moment at this point to discuss the use of *bifocal lenses*. Many stricken individuals seem to do one of two things. They may wear the glasses but strongly resist any ambulation that is not absolutely necessary for vital personal needs. Other patients may refuse to wear the glasses at all, which, of course, reduces their attention to abstract activity. In any instance, the process of readjustment can be hampered severely, and resistance to any activity can become insurmountable if bifocals are used.

This kind of a problem had never entered my mind until after I had struggled for a number of years with the negative effect of such lenses. I resisted the use of stairways, and even refused to use them because it was almost impossible to maintain any reasonable balance in either ascending and descending. I also failed to follow through on some of the physical therapy activities designed to maintain the remaining controls of body movement. I'm sure that my interest in reading waned because of the extreme difficulty I found in the use of these bifocal lenses. Not until some time after I started work on this manuscript did it occur to me that I should make a real investigation into the matter. At long last I found a congenial professional listener who really heard what I was trying to tell him, rather than recalling only the words he had seen in his texts. The bifocals were removed and replaced by two pairs of glasses, one for reading and one for ambulation. This too became a problem—but far less than that experienced with bifocals. My balance improved beyond my fondest hopes, and my deskwork became more efficient when I found it easier to concentrate on written materials.

The major problem in the slow recovery of my reading seemed to reside in the confusing glassline of the bifocals rather than in a weakened level of printed comprehension. A vast majority of other patients with a similar problem have revealed an obvious improvement in their reading activities after obtaining appropriate pairs of glasses. The retention span is highly dependent on the ease with which these patients can approach the reading chore. It seems so obvious now, but few clinicians seem to be able to discern the obvious. We must be sure that our patient can focus with relative ease before we make any attempt to estimate his ability to interpret printed material. At best, the printed word is abstract, so be realistic in your demands and hopes.

It is quite apparent that not all patients were wearing glasses prior to their accident. This does not mean, however, that they were not in need of them. Nor does it mean that they will not need them after their accident. When the motor and sensory tracts are involved elsewhere in the body, it is also possible for the controls of eye muscles to be affected. Hemionopsia is frequently present. Share your suspicions of possible damage with his doctor and ask for a specific evaluation before submitting the patient to the stress of visual concentration. When the client is having trouble following a line of print, keeping place in his reading, and is deficient in matching forms, letters, pictures, and words, it may be due to optical muscle imbalance rather than severe dysphasia for the printed word. It is first a medical problem that neither you nor the optometrist are capable of rectifying by yourselves. There is no room for careless assumptions in this mammoth problem of multiple disruptions.

Is Typing Feasible?

The vast majority of clients will have no need for the typewriter. Most of them have rarely used one since taking a course in high school. Typing is an extremely abstract activity, even more so than writing. Problems in vision often interfere with the act, and most patients really can't afford to purchase a typewriter. There are rare instances, however, when certain persons can return to their former employment as a typist. If so, seek the assistance of a teacher in the schools and follow her directions for practice in your center. There are a few books available, one of which is entitled, *Type with One Hand*.[1] Acquire this for your clinic library and have your patient take it to his teacher. Patients who have enough abstract ability can learn to type accurately and even as rapidly as a person with two hands. Had I known about this manual when I started this treatise, much time, energy, and frustration could have been altered.

The keyboard alphabet can be a meaningful aid in the recovery of spelling and letter recognition. In typing there is a need for sequencing the individual letters; consequently a latent script dysphasia may be modified. Aside from this specific usage, however, I strongly question the feasibility of any alphabet instruction.

Again, let me stress the fact that we are considering adults who already have memory problems for *useful* activities. Saying the alphabet is of no value when vital expressions are not forthcoming. Each letter is a word, so to speak, is it not? (A — eI), (B — bi), (C — si), (F — ɛf), (J — dʒeI), (L — ɛl), (M — ɛm), (P — pi), (Q — kju), (W — dʌblju), (X — ɛks), and (Y — waI), for a few examples. Sounding out words can be immediately rewarding, but the production of individual letters is terribly demoralizing, particularly when paralysis exists in half of the tongue and lips. Did you learn to speak by learning the alphabet? Confine its use to writing activities only and then only when absolutely imperative. You'll probably spend little time at it, if any, if you consider your patient's real needs.

[1] Richardson, Nina K., *Type with One Hand*, 2nd Ed., 1959. Write to South-Western Publishing Co., Cincinnati 27, Chicago 5, Dallas 2, San Francisco 3, or New Rochelle, N.Y., The Library of Congress Catalogue Card No. is 59-13366. The price is $1.17.

Severe Dysarthria

Be careful! The patients and their neurologists are your best advisors when it comes to motor and sensory deficits. When a sensory loss dominates, it is unlikely that you can do anything to improve articulation, and if motor recovery is *nil,* nothing can be done to speed up the process. Training for clarity should be one of the very last steps in your rehabilitative efforts. These patients have enough anxiety due to their lack of an appropriate vocabulary. Until it increases sufficiently, there is no time for concern about the beauty of articulation. Give the neurological tracts time to regenerate—if they can. Most patients improve without our pressures.

Some individuals have some functional carry-over of dysarthria, particularly if they have had little stimulation to rectify it over an extensive period of time. *One* of the best means for detecting this is through the use of nonsense syllables. An /s/ sound, for example, may be lateralized in habitual articulation. Initially, when severe paralysis reigns, tongue adjustments are impossible. Motor and sensory recovery is very gradual, and consequently faulty tongue placement can become subconsciously habitual, regardless of neurological improvements. When new phonetic contexts are introduced, the lateral emission of the /s/ sound is apt to disappear, that is (isi), (æsæ), (usu), etc. This is often easily detected, and the patient's correction of his running speech may follow automatically in many instances.

Frequently a slowing down in the rate of utterance will rectify sluggish productions. Rapidity of speech for the dysphasic is impossible with even a slight degree of paralysis. Most patients show a significant decrease in their rate of utterance, and very few can recover the pretraumatic speed of articulation. Our best assistance for them is indirect stimulation. Any anxiety increases spastic tension through the side of the damaged pathways from head to toe. The harder these patients try to relax their movements, the tighter the muscles become. The same is true in variations of speed: the faster they try to move, the slower they become. When this occurs, the resulting anxiety creates more tension and often results in withdrawal from clinical activity. Don't forget that they *want* to improve their functioning. This alone is pressure enough.

Most patients will eventually ask for help when they are ready for it. They know how they feel, and most often they use good judgment in their attempts to improve. Casual reminders are more effective than strong and unyielding commands and directions. These people are still human beings, so give them a right to behave that way!

Vocal intensity is largely based on respiratory control. I am not a physician, and there is little for me to discuss other than to plead for understanding the chore of breathing that the dysphasic person experiences. When the phonation is weak, I seek the counsel of physical medicine and carefully follow the forthcoming directions. Basically, I feel that if the patient is getting enough air for survival he will probably acquire a sufficiency for voice production—if the vocal cords can approximate in vibratory closure. Even these adjustments vary with anxiety and fatigue. Any increase in spastic tension of the thorax, abdomen, or larynx can alter the volume of the voice. The more secure such a patient is, the better he will be able to breathe and to phonate. It is also when he is secure that he wants to be heard. You will find that most of your clients speak loudly and clearly enough after they know you well enough. In this respect, they are like most of us. Unless we are secure, we too tend to mumble and use a weak voice. Our clients have additional body problems, and the more they are pushed, the more they fail. We must follow medical advice, maintain kind behavioral insight, and offer *realistic* rewards for performance. Do you now wonder about your patient's lack of self-esteem? His frustrations? How extensive would your feelings be in his place? Who wouldn't cry when one's social existence is continuously threatened by unneeded clinical pressures? Your patients know they are weeping. Most of them need to weep when we blindly ignore their feelings.

There are no mass training methods applicable to neurologically impaired persons. It is bad enough to fail at home among close family members. No patient likes to advertise his failures even to people who have a similar disruption. For the most part, the only thing in common among these dysphasic individuals is some kind of disturbance in communication. There are so many variations that any single approach cannot possibly be applicable to every patient. Each person is competing with himself, and this is competition enough. The patient knows what he has been, and he never forgets it. Even your own interruptions will be devasting enough to him though you are the supportive post to which he clings. The patient has no need to show off his disability. There is really nothing worth showing to anyone, even to himself. Dimensions in intelligence, occupation, and social and familial interests are truly unmatchable matters.

Not one of us feels comfortable in displaying our body scars, skinny legs, paunchy midriffs, or even our pidgeon toes, and certainly we reject the public demonstration of our own anxieties. Most of all, we demand the right and freedom to select our own close associates. Must we be exhibited in groups?

> 20   For a contrasting view of group therapy with dysphasic persons see the references by Corbin (3) and Sheehan (18).

Our clients are not puppets. They are individuals and deserve as much right to be afforded their privacy and our courtesy as any surgical patient. To be compelled to see one's image in the eyes of other disordered patients does little to help acquire language. Facial paralyses are not the kinds of images that any of us enjoy watching. Imagine the extent of the demoralizing distraction that a group of such clients are often forced to endure in the name of group therapy. The frequency of temper outbursts often increases, and this in itself is disrupting. Any behavior is alarmingly contagious. When they weep they do not weep alone, and the experience can be humiliating. Our major purpose should be that of assisting them to adjust to the majority of the population—not to other dysphasics, Surely if they cannot profit from the clinician's language stimulation, they will learn little from each other's inadequacies. Don't waste their limited energies by making them submit to these group sessions. Some of my colleagues have suggested that many of their clients need to see that they are doing better than others with dysphasia. My response is this: How about those who are doing worse? Moreover, few dysphasics can recognize that they are superior to anyone. If rarely they do realize that they are superior, their exaggerated compassion for the fellow patient dampens their appreciation of their own successes and creates negative identification instead. Don't group these patients in the hope that they will stimulate each other toward recovery.

THE FREQUENCY AND EXTENT OF CLINICAL VISITS

Keep the family aware of the vital importance of medical care. It is easy to forget the physician when the patient is free of negative health episodes. It will do no harm if the clinician sends a short summary to the patient's physician every six weeks or so. Much of what you observe is often helpful to him, and he too will better understand your recognition of a need for medical impressions. These patients and their families have to be helped to live within neurological limitations, seizures, hypertension, or arteriosclerotic disease. More than anyone else, the physician can help the patient, family, and you to stay within the bounds of the illness. These boundaries should guide your own clinical decisions. Mind and body are not separate entities, so arrange clinical appointments accordingly.

Frequency

The number of visits depends on the thoroughness with which familial insights can be obtained. In many instances, the recovery of language proceeds no faster than language acquired during infancy. The more successful you are with familial education, counseling, and guidance, the less often you will need to see the patient. He can have far more stimulation and need for language in a good home environment than in any clinical facility. Biweekly contacts with family members, for the first month to six weeks, should have precedence over frequent appointments with the patients.

The number of visits per week depends on the patient's over-all health and energies. We must also bear in mind that many patients' husbands or wives must maintain their employment, and this will also dictate the frequency of visits. From an ideal viewpoint, daily contact is most effective during the first month of enrollment. This not only assists in lessening the patient's reduced memory span, but it also aids his family to raise the pertinent questions that may otherwise be forgotten. The family members under such a regime seem to demonstrate clinical insights much more quickly and provide earlier assistance for their patient at home.

A gradual decrease in clinic visits is in order after you are satisfied that improved household insights are relatively stable. By the end of the second month, weekly appointments with the patient should suffice, but keep your clinical door and phone open to the family group. If you do not hear from them, then place a call yourself. No one likes to feel isolated, and most people don't like to overburden professionals with "silly questions." Invite their inquiries and be certain to give them a chance to drop in at times other than those reserved for their loved one. Recovery of language usage is a slow and vacillating process, and there will be difficulties in getting together. The loss of effective communication is indeed demoralizing, particularly when the patient must make frequent and often useless trips to your clinic. The appointments should be appropriate to each patient's individual needs.

Always bear in mind that none of us is capable of judging the chaotic spells of intellectual disorganization or internal emotionality that occur at times. The closer dysphasics are to being normal, the more they recognize their insufficiencies; hence, the more we become obligated to maintain personal contacts with them. If we can be available when they need us, we can assist them to retain their gains and also to help them to accept their weaknesses. They will need to complain—even to weep occasionally—in a relatively objective and permissive environment. These persons have long been engulfed in dark pits of utter hopelessness. Even the most positive degree of self-confidence will have a shadow of negativism for years to come. How long should we make ourselves available? Only our clients can answer this. We can only make sure they know that we will be available should they feel a need for supportive counsel. A few moments of our time can save months of recuperative progress. Be their handkerchief, their wailing wall if they need you in that role, so they can save their courage for maximal social adjustments. But always be their trusted friend.

In conclusion, we wish to make clear that this book is only an introduction to the very complicated problem of dysphasia. We hope you have at least begun to understand it, but all of us, like you, have much to learn. Our massive research literature on dysphasia rests on a tiny knoll of factual information. Nevertheless, progress is truly continuous, and we must always be alert to new literature. The most appropriate closing for this book, therefore, seems to be—ETC.

bibliography

1. Bixby, L., "Comeback from a Brain Operation," *Harper's Magazine* (November, 1952), pp. 69-73.
2. Brain, R., *Speech Disorders, Aphasia, Apraxia and Agnosia* (Washington: Butterworth, Inc., 1961).
3. Corbin, N. L., "Group Speech Therapy for Motor Aphasia and Dysarthria," *Journal Speech and Hearing Disorders,* XVI (1951), 21-34.
4. Darley, F. L., *Diagnosis and Appraisal of Communication Disorders* (Englewood Cliffs, N.J.: Prentice-Hall, Inc., 1964).
5. Eisenson, J., "Aphasics: Observations and Tentative Conclusions," *Journal Speech Disorders,* XII (1947), 290-92.
6. ——, *Examining for Aphasia,* rev. ed. (New York: Psychological Corporation, 1954).
7. ——, "Prognostic Factors Related to Language Rehabilitation in Aphasic Patients," *Journal Speech Disorders,* XIV (1949), 262-64.
8. Hall, W. A., "Return from Silence—A Personal Experience," *Journal Speech and Hearing Disorders,* XXVI (1961), 174-77.
9. Keenan, J. S., "A Method for Eliciting Naming Behavior from Aphasic Patients," *Journal Speech and Hearing Disorders,* XXXI (1966), 261-66.
10. Klingbeil, G. M., "The Historical Background of the Modern Speech Clinic: Part II. Aphasia," *Journal Speech Disorders,* IV (1939), 267-84.
11. Nielson, J. M., *Agnosia, Apraxia, Aphasia* (New York: Harper and Row, Publishers, 1946).
12. Penfield, W., and L. Roberts, *Speech and Brain Mechanisms* (Princeton, N.J.: Princeton University Press, 1959).
13. Rose, R. H., "A Physician's Account of His Own Aphasia," *Journal Speech Disorders,* XIII (1938), 294-305.
14. Russell, W. R., and M. L. E. Espir, *Traumatic Aphasia* (New York: Oxford University Press, 1961).

15. Schuell, H. M., "A Reevaluation of the Short Examination for Aphasia," *Journal Speech and Hearing Disorders*, XXXI (1966), 137-47.

16. ———, "Auditory Impairment in Aphasia: Significance and Retraining Procedures," *Journal Speech and Hearing Disorders*, XVII (1952), 353-56.

17. ———, J. J. Jenkins, and E. Jimines-Pabon, *Aphasia In Adults* (New York: Harper and Row, Publishers, 1964).

18. Sheehan, V. M., "Techniques in the Management of Aphasics," *Journal Speech Disorders*, XIII (1948), 241-46.

19. Smith, M., "Teaching an Aphasic How to Write Again," *Journal of Clinical Psychology*, 3rd ed., IV (1948), 419-23.

20. Turnbloom, M., and J. S. Myers, "A Group Discussion with Families of Aphasic Patients," *Journal Speech and Hearing Disorders*, XVII (1952), 393-96.

21. Van Riper, C., "Speech Disorders," Chap. 11 in Berg, I. A., and L. A. Pennington, eds., *An Introduction to Clinical Psychology*, 3rd ed. (New York: Ronald Press, 1966), 344-54.

22. Weisenberg, T., and K. F. McBride, *Aphasia* (New York: Oxford University Press, 1935).

23. Wepman, J. M., *Recovery from Aphasia* (New York: Ronald Press, 1951).

24. ———, "The Organization of Therapy for Aphasia: I. The In-Patient Treatment Center," *Journal Speech and Hearing Disorders*, XII (1958), 405-9.

25. ———, "The Relationship Between Self-Correction and Recovery from Aphasia," *Journal of Speech and Hearing Disorders*, XXIII (1958), 302-5.

26. ———, and L. V. Jones, *Studies in Aphasia: An Approach to Testing* (Chicago: Education-Industry Service, 1961).

index

Date Due